MIGRAINES

Also in the Your Health Series:

MIGRAINES

MORE THAN A
HEADACHE

Elizabeth Leroux M.D., FRCPC
Foreword by Isabelle Maréchal
Translated by Barbara Sandilands

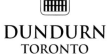

DUNDURN
TORONTO

Editor: Michael Melgaard
Design: Laura Boyle
Printer: Friesens
Cover Image: Fuse

Library and Archives Canada Cataloguing in Publication

Leroux, Elizabeth
[Migraine. English]

Migraines : more than a headache / Dr. Elizabeth Leroux, MD,
FRCBC ; foreword by Isabelle Maréchal ; translated by Barbara Sandilands.

(Your health)
Translation of: La migraine. Includes bibliographical references.
Issued in print and electronic formats.
ISBN 978-1-4597-3289-6 (paperback).-- ISBN 978-1-4597-3290-2 (pdf).-- ISBN 978-1-4597-3291-9 (epub)

1. Migraine. 2. Migraine--Treatment. I. Sandilands, Barbara, translator II. Title. III. Title: Migraine. English.

RC392.L4713 2016   616.8'4912   C2015-908065-7
                                                C2015-908066-5

1   2   3   4   5   20   19   18   17   16

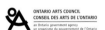

We acknowledge the support of the **Canada Council for the Arts** and the **Ontario Arts Council** for our publishing program.
We also acknowledge the financial support of the **Government of Canada** through the **Canada Book Fund** and **Livres Canada
Books**, and the **Government of Ontario** through the **Ontario Book Publishing Tax Credit** and the **Ontario Media Development
Corporation**.

Care has been taken to trace the ownership of copyright material used in this book. The author and the publisher welcome any
information enabling them to rectify any references or credits in subsequent editions.
— *J. Kirk Howard, President*

The publisher is not responsible for websites or their content unless they are owned by the publisher.

Printed and bound in Canada.

Visit us at
Dundurn.com | @dundurnpress | Facebook.com/dundurnpress | Pinterest.com/Dundurnpress

Dundurn
3 Church Street, Suite 500
Toronto, Ontario, Canada
M5E 1M2

To my mother, who showed me how to take care of others,
and to my father, who taught me the importance of trying to understand them.

Thank you to my family, my friends, my colleagues, my patients,
my students, my cats, my professors, my musical soulmates....
To all those I've met along the way, and who have helped me,
in a thousand ways, to write this book.

Table of Contents

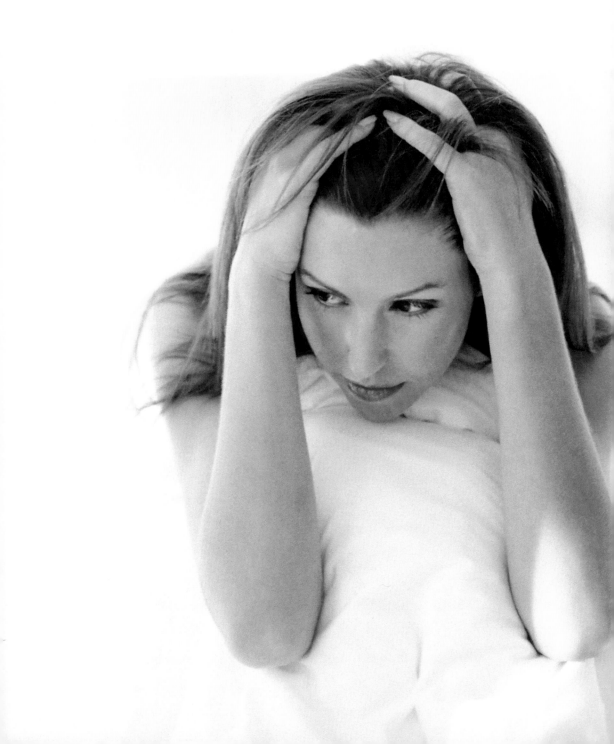

Foreword

When Dr. Elizabeth Leroux asked if I would write the foreword to her book, I was delighted to accept the opportunity to talk about the cross we migraine sufferers have to bear. How many times have I been told by a doctor who knew nothing about my condition, "It's all in your head, my dear!" How many times have I huddled under my sheets in the dark, powerless, asking myself who on earth was going to be able to rescue me from this black hole that's ruining my life?

I've had migraines for a very long time. Like a ritual that comes to haunt me, every November coincides with the return of severe attacks that plague me for several weeks. I'm no longer myself and my head feels like it's going to explode. I curse my brain, whose excess electricity causes me terrible pain. I'd give almost anything not to suffer like this. The increasing pain in my left eye, the temple that starts to throb and reverberates deep down in my skull. I have what are commonly known as chronic migraines, triggered by the season and my surroundings, among other things. There's no way I can avoid them. That's just the way it is. The attack can occur at any time. It's an incurable disease. I depend on triptans and, recently, on injections of DHE, which make me very nauseated. It's serious. My symptoms are the kind that are so painful they send you to the hospital — they're quite simply intolerable.

Every migraine sufferer deserves to be closely monitored by a neurologist. Mine completely changed my life. Dr. Michel Aubé is a pioneer in migraine treatment in Canada. When I met him a few years ago, I was experiencing full-blown rebound migraines; in other words, my migraines were caused by too many anti-migraine medications. The phenomenon is now well-known. I could have bought the company that manufactures Advil and Tylenol, I'd swallowed so many of them.

The worst thing is that you end up developing a kind of fear between attacks that the migraine will come back and overwhelm you again. That the army of soldiers with sledgehammers will return and turn your head into a minefield. For the brain of a migraine sufferer is a brain at war. The battle is fought at our expense. We're the powerless victims of a disease — but one that we can nonetheless manage to control somewhat by changing our lifestyle habits.

This has been a great revelation to me in the past few years. And Dr. Elizabeth Leroux confirms it in this book: people who get migraines, or should I say, women who get migraines, since the disease affects twice as many women as men, must not just resign themselves to suffering alone, silently, in the dark. They cannot rely solely on an uncaring healthcare system. They must first and foremost take charge of themselves. This means making changes.

Changing our lifestyle habits isn't easy to do, but the effort is worth it. I had to give up some foods, including dairy products and processed meats, and reduce caffeine and gluten intake. I eat smaller meals more often. And I now pay attention to my biological clock. When I'm tired, I sleep. I no longer fight my headaches. If I have to rest, I do.

You have to recognize your triggering factors and accept your particular condition. What really helped me was the support of my spouse, family, and friends, who were able to see and understand my distress, my pain, and my powerlessness. Being around migraineurs who are not ashamed to make their condition known also helps greatly. Don't be afraid to talk about it.

In this book, Dr. Leroux comes across as an invaluable ally. With a great deal of empathy, she describes to a lay audience the complex disease called migraine. Her lengthy experience with migraineurs makes her one of the rare specialists who will teach you how the brains of patients with this incurable disease function, a disease that can however be alleviated with monitoring and specific medications. Lastly, migraine sufferers will find here the explanations they've needed to understand their disease and to no longer feel they are controlled by it. For there are many of us who hope that one day this brain that causes us so much pain will settle down and allow us to lead a full and tranquil life.

Isabelle Maréchal

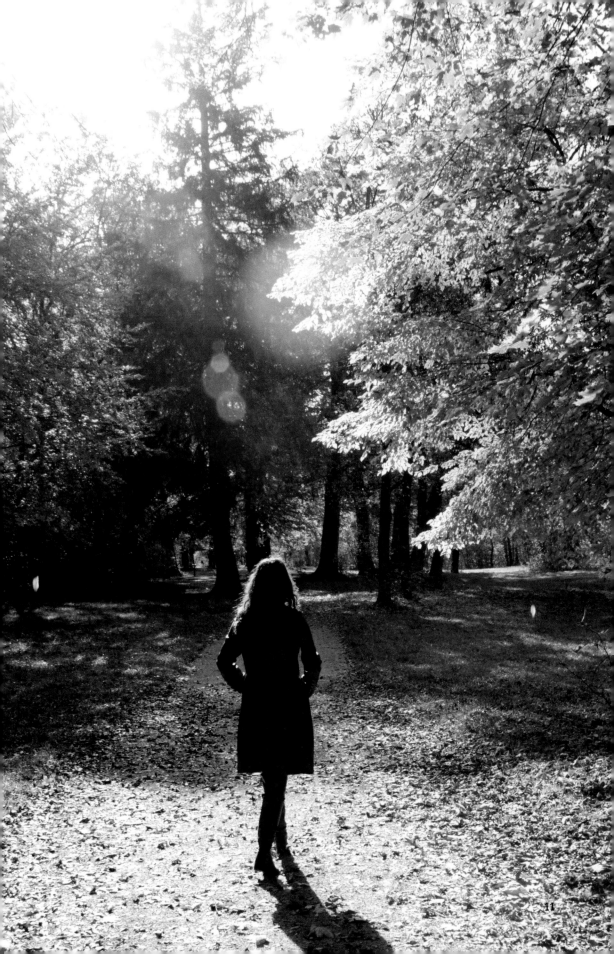

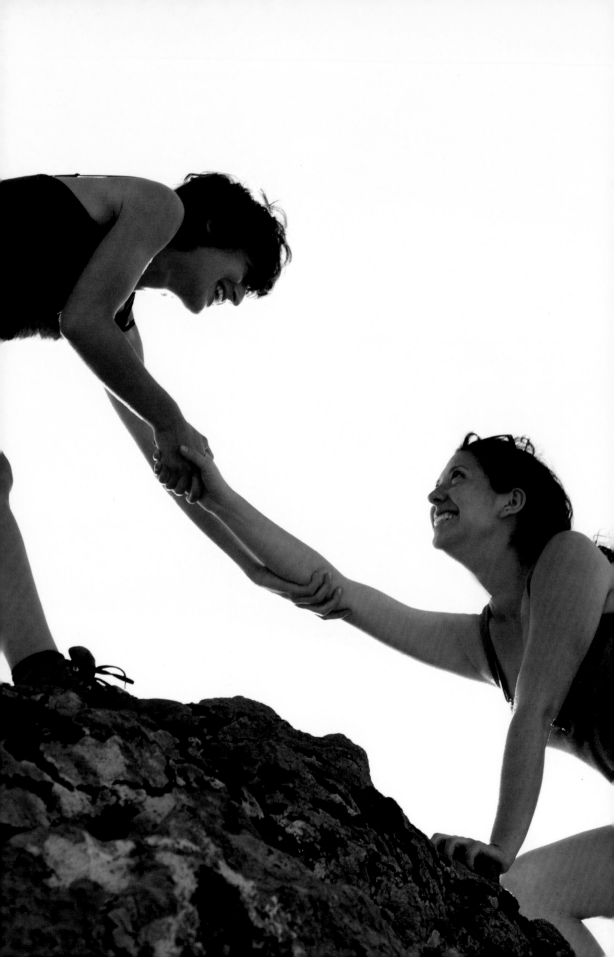

Understand More, Live Better

According to the World Health Organization, migraine is the third most common disease in the world, in all categories, after dental caries and tension-type headaches. That shows you just how common headaches are! Most people will have a headache at one time or another. However, migraine is not an ordinary headache.

When I first began dealing with migraine sufferers, I was struck by a common element in their stories: for years, they had faced a lack of understanding from their friends and family, their employers, and even their doctors. No one believed them when they talked about their symptoms, about the intolerable pain, the unbearable light, the irritating noises, their inability to function during an attack. In my office, I listened to hundreds of accounts and real-life stories. I heard about the countless disappointments: ruined trips, missed anniversaries, hours spent in front of the computer with nausea, weight gain caused by taking drugs, failure of treatments, numerous consultations only to be told there's nothing wrong with you, the accusing look of an employer after another day of sick leave. I witnessed teary outbursts when I explained to these people, after they had lived through years of guilt and solitude, internal battles, and soul-searching, that they had a real disease. That they were neither crazy, nor lazy, nor faking it. And, most important, that there

might be something that could be done to help them. My favourite sentence was: I don't promise I'll succeed, but I promise I'll try. Because in order to get better, you at least have to try.

Migraine is a neurological disease, a problem in the brain. It's complex, it has many faces, and its mechanisms are still poorly understood. But it exists. It's real. And it's the seventh-ranked cause of disability worldwide, again according to the World Health Organization. It keeps people from functioning and is the cause of a great deal of suffering. I've been able to see this suffering in my office. And part of the agony felt by all of these patients did not stem from the migraine itself, but rather from the perception of this disease. Denial, passivity, blame, disbelief, disparagement, even jokes in poor taste. We don't yet have a treatment to cure migraine, but we can at the very least change our perception of the disease and stop doing harm to those who have it by refusing to recognize their symptoms. To change our perception, destroy taboos, and deconstruct myths, we have to explain it to people, we have to educate them. We have to help people understand. And understanding a neurological problem like this one is quite a challenge.

This is the challenge I'm trying to meet by writing this book. By presenting scientific knowledge in lay terms, I'll outline what we in the medical community know, so that migraine sufferers and those close to them can also understand this disease. The book's first objective is therefore to explain what migraine is in order to have it recognized as a real health problem that deserves consideration and care.

Aside from taboos, migraineurs face another significant difficulty. No pill can cure migraine. The brain of a migraine sufferer is influenced by the environment and by lifestyle habits. People with migraines have to make decisions every month, every week, even every day, that might affect their daily routine, whether at work or in their personal

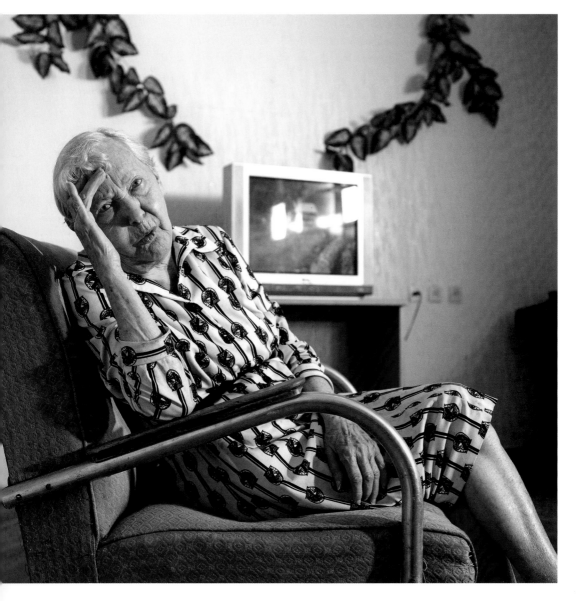

lives. To make these decisions, they have to become their own experts, know themselves, and learn about treatments, triggers, things to avoid, which habits to adopt. Migraineurs have to learn to live with migraine. They have to learn self-management.

In an era when the health system is under pressure, professionals have little time to educate their patients. Since migraine is not a public health priority, few resources are allocated to help multi-disciplinary teams. Access to specialized clinics is limited, and the waiting lists are long. The second objective of this book is therefore to give men and women who suffer from migraine tools to help them take charge of themselves and get the most out of their treatments.

I hope this book helps make known the reality experienced by people with migraine and encourages us all to mobilize to ensure better care, break down myths, and promote research.

Happy reading!

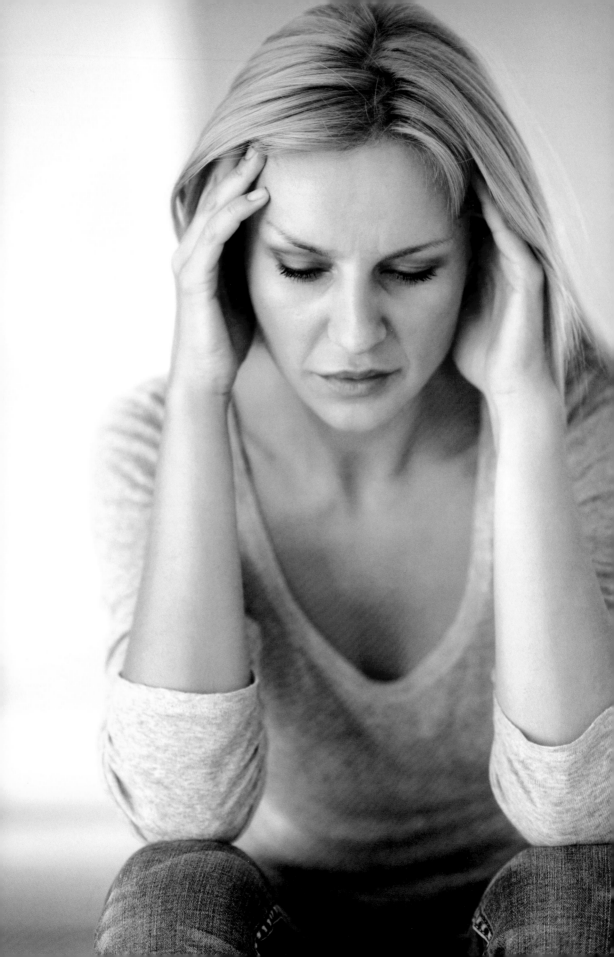

CHAPTER 1

Migraine or Headache?

There is only one cardinal rule:
One must always listen to the patient.
— OLIVER SACKS

Headache is one of the most common symptoms doctors see and one of the most difficult to evaluate. A headache may be caused by a great many medical factors, from meningitis, to the intake of certain drugs, to sleep apnea. The International Classification of Headache Disorders includes more than two hundred possible diagnoses grouped in categories (Figure 2)!

DIAGNOSING HEADACHES

THE MEDICAL QUESTIONNAIRE
Doctors nowadays have access to an impressive arsenal of diagnostic tests — blood tests, scanners, magnetic resonance imaging, electroencephalograms — but in the headache world, the most useful tools remain the questionnaire and the physical examination. The description provided by the patient is vital, as headache is a subjective symptom impossible to measure in the blood or with an electrophysiological test.

Only patients can give doctors the clues that will lead them to the right diagnosis (Figure 1). The first consultation for a headache disorder may be lengthy if the case is complex, the problem goes back several years, there is more than one kind of headache, or the cause of the pain is hard to identify. In a typical migraine situation, where there are no other health problems, the patient's history can be covered very quickly, and the doctor can immediately focus on managing the attacks.

PRIMARY OR SECONDARY HEADACHES
Primary headaches, caused by a nervous system dysfunction with no visible lesions or associated disease, are usually distinguished from secondary headaches, caused by visible lesions on the head or neck, or by metabolic disorders in the organism. Since brain function resembles that of a computer, the distinction between primary and secondary headaches can be illustrated by an example from the world of computing.

MEDICAL HISTORY

Topics to Discuss During a Medical Consultation

Topic	Examples	
General State of Health		
PERSONAL MEDICAL HISTORY	Medical history, operations, accidents, dental problems, psychiatric disorders.	Some diseases may be associated with headaches, either as cause or effect.
FAMILY HISTORY	History of migraine, epilepsy, neurological disease in the family, especially in the first degree.	Some kinds of headaches are hereditary.
LIFESTYLE HABITS	Sleep, coffee consumption, smoking, alcohol, exercise, work, children, stress management.	Adapting lifestyle habits is essential.
Headache History		
NUMBER OF HEADACHES	Do you have different types of headaches?	It's best to focus on the pain that bothers you most, but other kinds of pain also have to be taken into account.
DURATION OF THE PROBLEM	Is the headache recent or is it a headache you've had for many years that has just gotten worse?	A genuinely new headache may need to be investigated. The history of migraine may go back to childhood.
HEADACHE FREQUENCY	Do you have attacks interspersed with normal days or do you instead have very frequent or even continual pain?	The approach is very different depending on whether individual attacks or ongoing headaches are the problem.
LENGTH OF ATTACKS	When you have attacks, do they last seconds? Minutes? Hours? Days?	It's sometimes hard to determine the duration of attacks if they are frequent and combined with a background headache.
LOCATION	Is the pain on one side? Both? In the forehead? In the neck? In the eye?	Even if the location doesn't always result in a diagnosis, it's important information.
TYPE OF PAIN	Do you feel pressure? Throbbing? An electric shock or burning sensation?	Some of the pain's characteristics can influence treatment, especially in the case of neuralgias.

FIGURE 1

Headache History (continued)

TRIGGERING AND AGGRAVATING FACTORS	Alcohol, foods, exercise, coughing, sexual activity, stress, lack of sleep.	Some triggers are especially associated with migraines, while others point to other causes.
ACCOMPANYING SYMPTOMS	Nausea, difficulty tolerating sound and light, tinnitus, neck pain, watery eyes, etc.	Although certain symptoms are more common in migraine sufferers, they may be present in other diseases as well.
NEUROLOGICAL SYMPTOMS	Problems with vision, language, strength, memory sensation, and balance.	The presence of neurological symptoms is worrying and warrants an investigation.
GENERAL SYMPTOMS	Fever, weight loss, feeling generally unwell.	When general health is affected this is of concern and warrants an investigation.
IMPACT ON FUNCTIONING	Employment status, disability, difficulties in accomplishing daily or personal tasks.	Whatever their cause, headaches can impair daily functioning. This aspect is often overlooked.

Medication History

CURRENT MEDICATIONS	Medications used for headaches, but also for other medical disorders.	Always bring a complete, up-to-date list with you. Some medications can cause headaches.
PREVIOUS TRIAL TREATMENTS	Treatments for attacks, preventive treatments, and contraceptives.	Non-tolerated or ineffective medications must be permanently avoided. Doses are also important.
FREQUENCY OF CURRENT MEDICATION INTAKE	Use of painkillers and other medications for headaches or other kinds of pain.	Medication-overuse headache is a common problem treated by discontinuing the medication.

Conclusions and Expectations

ANYTHING TO ADD?	It's important to be sure that all the patient's headache-related concerns have been discussed.	Some of the patient's observations, worries, or perceptions can have an impact on treatment.
PATIENT EXPECTATIONS	The doctor doubtless has solutions to suggest, but the patient's hopes are sometimes different.	Patients suffering from headaches must take an active part in their treatment and participate in decision-making, in accordance with their priorities, knowledge, and concerns.

THE INTERNATIONAL CLASSIFICATION OF HEADACHE DISORDERS

	Category	Examples (non-exhaustive list)
1	Migraine	Includes the various kinds of migraine (with or without aura, episodic, chronic, prolonged attack).
2	Tension-Type Headache	Episodic or chronic tension-type headache, with or without pericranial tenderness.
3	Trigeminal Autonomic Cephalalgias	Cluster headache, paroxysmal or continuous hemicranias, SUNCT.
4	Other Primary Headache Disorders	Headaches caused by exertion, sexual activity, cough, new daily persistent headache (NDPH).
5	Headache Attributed to Trauma	Headaches attributed to cranial and cervical trauma, headache following brain surgery.
6	Headache Attributed to Cervical Vascular Disorder	Headache following a stroke, aneurism, cerebral hemorrhage, blood clot.
7	Headache Attributed to Non-Vascular Intracranial Disorder	Brain tumours, intracranial hypertension or hypotension, headaches attributed to epilepsy.
8	Headache Attributed to a Substance or Its Withdrawal	Medication overuse (triptans, narcotics), caffeine withdrawal, estrogen pill withdrawal. Several medications.
9	Headache Attributed to Brain Infection	Meningitis, brain abscess, bacteria, viruses, parasites.
10	Headache Attributed to a Metabolic Disorder	Sleep apnea, scuba diving, hypothyroidism, high altitude, hypertension, and other causes.
11	Headache Attributed to a Disorder of the Neck, Eyes, Teeth, Ears	Cervicogenic headache, sinusitis, temporomandibular disorder, glaucoma, dental disorders.
12	Headache Attributed to Psychiatric Disorder	Somatization and psychotic disorders.
13	Painful Cranial Neuropathies and Other Facial Pains	Trigeminal neuralgia, occipital (or Arnold's) neuralgia, stomatopyrosis (or burning mouth syndrome), facial pain attributed to multiple sclerosis.
14	Other	Headache with cause unknown or not elsewhere classified.
A	Appendix	Headaches as yet unclassified.

FIGURE 2   *International Classification of Headache Disorders 3.*

If a computer doesn't function, it may be because of a software problem (the program is defective or infected with a computer virus, but the device is not damaged) or a hardware problem (the hard disk is damaged, the fan is broken, and the device has overheated). Software problems represent primary headaches, such as migraine and tension-type headaches, and hardware problems represent secondary headaches, such as meningitis and brain tumours (Figure 3).

Most people who go to see a doctor for a headache disorder have primary headaches that are most often migraine (Figure 4), but even though migraine is the most common diagnosis, all other causes must nonetheless be initially ruled out!

DIAGNOSES MADE IN A HEADACHE CLINIC

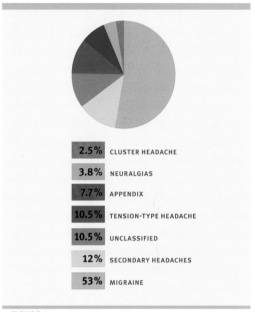

2.5%	CLUSTER HEADACHE
3.8%	NEURALGIAS
7.7%	APPENDIX
10.5%	TENSION-TYPE HEADACHE
10.5%	UNCLASSIFIED
12%	SECONDARY HEADACHES
53%	MIGRAINE

FIGURE 4   Adapted from Pedraza, *Neurologia*, 2014.

VISIBLE LESION, INVISIBLE DYSFUNCTION

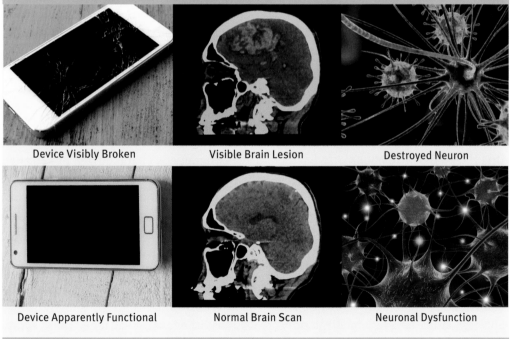

Device Visibly Broken   Visible Brain Lesion   Destroyed Neuron

Device Apparently Functional   Normal Brain Scan   Neuronal Dysfunction

FIGURE 3

Warning Signs

The first thing to check when evaluating someone with headaches is whether there are any warning signs; this can be done using the SNOOP mnemonic (Figure 5). If there are other symptoms, such as fever, weight loss, or a disease that lowers immunity (cancer or the AIDS virus), a more in-depth investigation is required. If the neurological examination is abnormal, or if the person reports neurological symptoms (disorders related to vision, language, strength, sensation, balance, memory), brain imaging is called for. The risk of having a disease other than migraine increases with age; this is why the level of concern with regard to people over fifty is high. Some headaches occur suddenly and are sometimes described as thunderclap headaches. This kind of pain rings alarm bells, and the doctor will immediately suspect a hemorrhage caused by an aneurism or a number of other causes, including brain artery disease. If the headache is gradually getting worse from day to day, or is perhaps worse when the person is lying down and is accompanied by nausea, the doctor will suspect intracranial hypertension, possibly caused by a brain tumour.

Do I Have a Brain Tumour?

Most people suffering from an unaccustomed headache will be afraid they have a brain tumour. Everybody seems to have a neighbour or cousin who has received this kind of catastrophic diagnosis. Many patients worry when their doctor doesn't prescribe a brain scan after a headache consultation. But brain tumours are actually very rare and are only responsible for a very small minority of headaches. The risk of finding a brain tumour during a visit to a general practitioner for

headache is one in a thousand, and most of these tumours are benign. Furthermore, 85 percent of patients with a brain tumour will have other symptoms besides headache, and their physical examination will be abnormal in the vast majority of cases. The risk of a brain tumour is higher in people over fifty and in young children. Usually the headache will have occurred in recent weeks and will have become increasingly intense. A headache that's been there for years is not usually caused by a brain tumour.

DIAGNOSING MIGRAINES

If you have recurring headaches, it's very possible you have migraines without knowing it. Two-thirds of migraine sufferers are actually not diagnosed (Figure 6). Obviously, some of them are not bothered very much by their migraines and don't go to see a doctor. Others do, but their attacks are moderate and assumed to be tension-type headaches. In some cases, even when the migraine attacks are obvious and keep the person from functioning normally, a diagnosis is never made (see the account on page 26), preventing proper care from being provided.

Migraine is characterized by repeated attacks interspersed with intervals when the person functions more or less normally. These attacks usually have typical characteristics (Figures 7 and 8) that also help distinguish them from the tension-type headache described a little later in this chapter. Migraine is a complex neurological disorder comprising many symptoms other than headache. These symptoms and their biological mechanisms are discussed in greater detail in Chapter 3.

WARNING SIGNS ASSOCIATED WITH HEADACHES

S	**Systemic Signs or Symptoms**	Weight loss, use of immunosuppressants, history of cancer, HIV, etc.
N	**Neurological Signs or Symptoms**	Papillary edema, hemiparesis (weakness on one side), diplopia (double vision), dysarthria (language problems), etc.
O	Onset, How It Occurs	Sudden or gradual headache.
O	Older, the Patient's Age	New headache after fifty.
P	Previous Progressive Postural	Headache different from usual pain (previous). Gradual, gets worse. Postural, varies depending on whether the person is standing up or lying down.

FIGURE 5   D.W. Dodick, *Adv Stud Med*, 2003.

Obviously, migraine sufferers may also have tension-type headaches as well as their "real migraines." That said, headache specialists often observe that migraineurs themselves wrongly describe their more moderate migraines as tension-type headaches.

WHY DIDN'T THE DOCTOR PRESCRIBE A SCAN?

If there are no warning signs, given a typical migraine history and a normal neurological examination, there is usually no reason for brain imaging. This approach is recommended by several national neurological associations. Despite this, many doctors require radiological tests with no justification. In Switzerland, 84 percent of doctors automatically prescribe cerebral magnetic resonance imaging following a headache consultation. The main reason for doing so is the desire to reassure their patient. Many doctors are also trying to guard against any malpractice lawsuits. A doctor will never be blamed for having prescribed a useless test.

But here's the problem — the more you look, the more you find! Several studies have shown that when brain scans are carried out on healthy volunteers, abnormalities will be found in 2 to 5 percent of them, most with no impact on health. Thus, in trying to reassure patients, there's a risk of worrying them more by finding a benign abnormality likely unrelated to the headache. What's more, given the very high incidence of headaches, unjustified investigations represent a significant cost for the healthcare system. In an era when the public system is under pressure and access to imaging is limited, doctors and patients must ask themselves if it's reasonable to prescribe useless tests with the sole aim of better reassuring patients and protecting doctors from malpractice suits. It must also be stressed that telling migraine sufferers they have "nothing" is not very productive in terms of future care. A migraine diagnosis should lead to a process of educating the patient and prescribing appropriate treatments.

MIGRAINE DIAGNOSIS: THE TIP OF THE ICEBERG

	MEN	WOMEN
Diagnosed	29 %	41%
Undiagnosed	71 %	59%

FIGURE 6 — R.B. Lipton et al., *Arch Intern Med*, 1992.

MIGRAINE AND HEADACHE: SUMMARY

	Migraine	Tension-type headache
UNILATERAL	+	o
PULSATILE	+	o
INTENSITY	Moderate to severe	Light to moderate
WORSENED BY EXERCISE	+	o
NAUSEA	+	o
PHOTO- OR PHONOPHOBIA	Frequent	Sometimes
DURATION	From 4 to 72 hours	From 30 minutes to 7 days

FIGURE 7 — Elizabeth Leroux.

OFFICIAL DIAGNOSTIC CRITERIA FOR MIGRAINE

A	At least five attacks fulfilling criteria B-D.	A first episode of headache cannot be diagnosed as a migraine.
B	Headache attacks lasting four to seventy-two hours, untreated or unsuccessfully treated.	A migraine may last less than four hours if it's effectively treated.
C	Headache has at least two of the following four characteristics: 1. unilateral location; 2. pulsating quality; 3. moderate or severe pain intensity; 4. aggravation by or causing avoidance of routine physical activity.	These characteristics are not essential. Some migraines are bilateral and not pulsatile — hence the possibility of two out of four characteristics.
D	At least one of the following two characteristics: 1. nausea and/or vomiting; 2. photophobia and phonophobia.	These symptoms are often associated with migraines, but may also occur with other kinds of headache.
E	Not better accounted for by another diagnosis.	Secondary headache must be excluded, especially when there are warning signs.

FIGURE 8 — Adapted from ICHD-3.

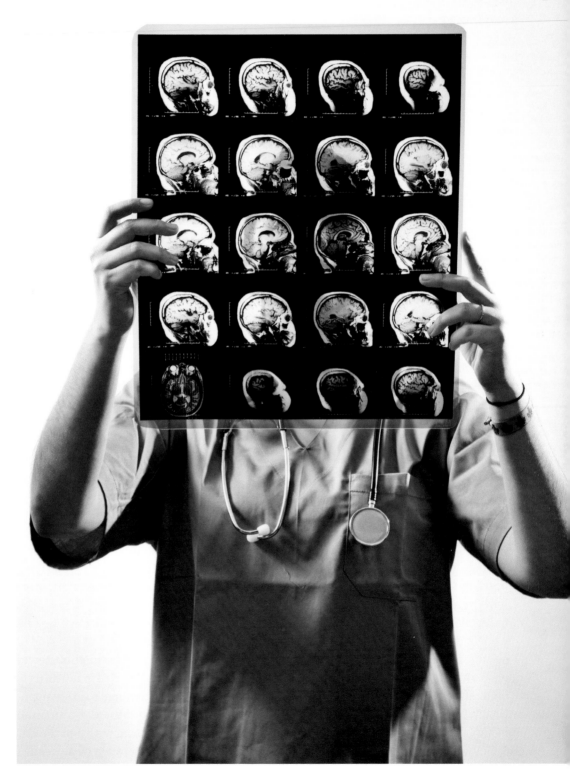

"RECURRENT SINUSITIS"

According to a study carried out by the Mayo Clinic in the United States, 75 percent of people with "sinus headaches" actually suffer from migraines, as revealed by a detailed questionnaire. The diagnostic confusion stems from the fact that these people feel pain in their forehead and maxillary sinuses, and experience nasal congestion during the attacks. They may also get migraines in response to sinus irritants (allergies, head cold). It's possible therefore for sinusitis to trigger a migraine, but it's also possible for a migraine to be so much like sinusitis that you can't tell them apart!

Nancy, 39

When she was eight, Nancy started to have migraines. As a teenager, she sometimes had to miss school during the worst attacks. In a discussion with her pediatrician, it was explained to her that school was no doubt a source of stress for her. One day, in her twenties, she had to go to emergency. Over the years, she had eight brain scans and always got the same response: "Your scan is normal; there's nothing wrong with you." Nancy did not understand how there could be nothing wrong, when she would still have intense pain attacks accompanied by vomiting. One day, a family doctor who himself had migraines sent her to a neurologist. Today, Nancy understands her condition better and has ways of more effectively managing her attacks. Finally, she knows the problem is not "all in her head."

OTHER DIAGNOSES

Arriving at a diagnosis for headaches is not always easy. Patients may relate vague or varying case histories. Furthermore, different kinds of headaches have similarities; it's therefore very important to collect the details so as to be able to tell them apart.

TENSION-TYPE HEADACHES: THE COMMON HEADACHE

The tension-type headache is the second most common disease in the world! Between 20 and 50 percent of people will have a tension-type headache at one time or other. While this type of headache is very common in the population, it results in far fewer visits to the doctor than migraine, which impacts daily life in a much more severe way (Figure 9). The "little run-of-the-mill headache, the kind everyone gets" is not too disturbing and rarely requires a visit to the doctor. The pain is often diffuse, felt on both sides of the head, and is not accompanied by nausea or difficulty tolerating noise and light. It's not a throbbing pain and, most often, non-prescription painkillers are enough to relieve it. Cases of chronic continuous tension-type headache are very rare.

It's surprising to note that such a common ailment remains mysterious. Whereas our understanding of migraine is increasing, tension-type headaches resist researchers' efforts. It must be said that, given the weak impact of this kind of headache on how people function, fewer medical teams are interested in it. The term "tension" doesn't refer here to arterial tension, but instead to muscular or mental tension often associated with a particular event. A connection between what is called myofascial syndrome, or areas of excessive tension in the muscles, and tension-type headache is now recognized.

HORTON'S HEADACHE OR CLUSTER HEADACHE

Cluster headache is usually quite easy to recognize, as it's the most intense pain known to humans, even worse than childbirth, kidney stones, or amputation without anaesthesia. During these attacks, many patients consider suicide, to put an end once and for all to their fierce and intolerable pain — hence the term "suicide headache."

Cluster headaches are often centred on the eye or the temple, although the pain may radiate to the neck or teeth. They strike suddenly and are accompanied by visible symptoms: red and watery eyes, drooping eyelids, and runny nose. Sufferers tend to fidget and become agitated, stamp their feet, or even hit the wall to relieve the pain. There may be nausea, but less often than during a migraine attack. The attack lasts from thirty minutes to three hours, or sometimes longer if it isn't treated. Attacks may

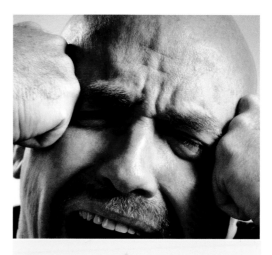

Paul, 42

"I remember my first attack very well. I'd never felt pain like that before. I thought I was going crazy! It felt like someone was stabbing a white-hot knife into my eye. After a few minutes, my eye started to water, and the pain spread to my temple and cheek. I didn't know what to do. My spouse tried to get close to me, but I didn't want her to touch me. I was ashamed of losing control like that. When the attack was over, I was exhausted. Two hours of sheer hell. And the next night, I had the same kind of attack. For two months, the attacks kept recurring. So I went to see an optometrist, who suspected something and sent me to a neurologist. I now use sumatriptan injectors to relieve the attacks."

MIGRAINE: LESS COMMON BUT MORE DISABLING THAN TENSION-TYPE HEADACHES

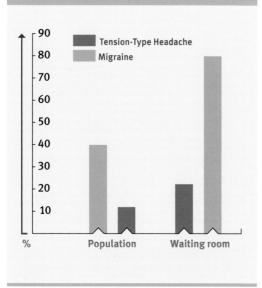

FIGURE 9   R.B. Lipton et al., *Neurology*, 2003.

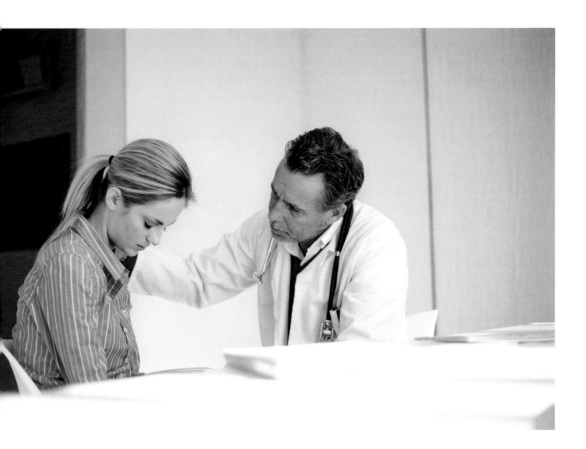

recur up to eight times a day, but on average frequency ranges from one attack every two days to three attacks a day. Cluster attacks tend to occur at specific times and during specific periods of the year. For several weeks or several months, attacks will occur regularly, and then they may stop for months or even years. They are often triggered by drinking alcohol.

The cause of cluster headache is the subject of major research. The area of the brain key to the onset of these attacks is likely the hypothalamus, the structure responsible, among other functions, for wake-sleep cycles and endocrine regulation. If you think you have cluster headache, you should consult a doctor and will likely be sent to see a neurologist. Treatments exist, both to alleviate attacks and to prevent

them. More recently, neurostimulation approaches, such as intracranial and occipital neurostimulation, have proven to be effective in the most severe cases.

TRIGEMINAL NEURALGIA

Trigeminal neuralgia, or TGN, is not really a headache, but rather facial pain that feels like an electric shock in the cheek, jaw, or teeth. This disorder most often affects the elderly, but is also seen in younger people. The pain is sometimes caused by touching a sensitive or trigger area. These areas may be in the mouth or on the face, often around the lips or on the edge of the nose. Depending on the severity of the disease, the shocks may be very frequent or occur only if the trigger area is touched. TGN is sometimes caused by contact between an artery and the trigeminal nerve, in the brain stem. When it throbs, the artery may irritate the nerve, causing the shocks.

It's not always easy to tell the difference between neuralgia caused by a disorder inside the brain and neuralgia caused by a dental problem. Some patients have had their teeth extracted in hopes of curing neuralgia that was in fact caused by an artery pressing on the trigeminal nerve! A dental procedure without complications may uncover trigeminal neuralgia — the stimulation of the nerve during the procedure reveals a more deep-rooted disorder that hadn't yet been noticed. This kind of disorder requires close collaboration between dentist and neurologist to choose appropriate treatments and avoid unnecessary and even harmful procedures.

As it progresses, TGN often goes through more active phases interspersed with remissions. Sometimes, during these exacerbations, those affected can neither eat nor speak, as the slightest movement of the face triggers intolerable shocks. This causes great anxiety and may cause sleeplessness, making the pain worse. A TGN attack can be a medical emergency. To stabilize the condition, several medications are used. In some cases, surgical procedures are recommended.

POST-TRAUMATIC HEADACHE

Life is not always a long and tranquil river! From the child who falls off a bicycle to the car driver who has an accident and the athlete injured on the field, there's no lack of examples of head trauma.

In the big family of headaches, we might say that post-traumatic headache is the elephant in the room: a huge problem no one seems to notice — one that everyone sees but nobody talks about. Following head trauma or a "whiplash" caused when a vehicle they were riding in stops suddenly, many people will experience post-traumatic syndrome: headaches, sleep disorders, irritability, difficulties concentrating, dizziness, etc. An avalanche of sometimes incapacitating symptoms can result, which are subjective and hard to measure with tests. Post-traumatic syndrome tends to diminish over time, but a significant percentage of people will continue to have headaches and neck pain, sometimes permanently. Several scenarios are possible: if the person who suffered the trauma had migraines previously, the trauma may trigger more frequent migraines and they may become chronic, with very frequent attacks interspersed with less intense headaches. A new kind of headache may also develop and be added to or combine with pre-existing headaches.

Post-traumatic headache can take many forms. The pain may be located anywhere. It may resemble a migraine or a tension-type headache, and it may even include electric shocks reminiscent of neuralgia. It may also be accompanied by dizziness and persistent difficulties in concentrating. The cause of all of this? Recent studies have highlighted abnormalities in the brain networks, the delicate connections that link our neurons together and allow our brain to function normally. This is called a diffuse axonal injury and is very hard to see without specialized technology.

Despite its high prevalence and significant social cost, until just recently post-traumatic headache was the forgotten headache in clinical research. No treatment has yet been tested specifically for this disease in high-quality studies. As a result, doctors will usually try a multidisciplinary approach for neck problems (physiotherapy, osteopathy, injections in the joints of the neck) and prescribe medications studied for migraines, sometimes successfully. In recent years, research teams have been focusing on post-traumatic headaches in soldiers and athletes, which should advance the body of knowledge.

IDIOPATHIC INTRACRANIAL HYPERTENSION (PSEUDOTUMOR CEREBRI)

This disease is caused by an increase in pressure inside the skull. It often occurs in overweight women, without our knowing exactly why, as the vast majority of obese women do not have this disorder. Children may be affected by it. The headache is often diffuse, is worse in the morning, and gets worse when the person bends over. Slight nausea is sometimes experienced. Intracranial pressure compresses the optic nerve and may cause the visual field to shrink. The compression of other nerves may result in double vision, a symptom that should always justify an urgent medical visit. A diagnosis of this medical condition is made using brain imaging (the presence of a tumour that would increase pressure has to be excluded) and a spinal tap to measure pressure. The cause of pseudotumor cerebri is still poorly understood, but there is definitely a disruption of the mechanisms controlling intracranial pressure. Treatment revolves around weight loss, but certain drugs are also used. Sometimes repeated spinal taps are done to drain the cerebrospinal fluid and decrease pressure.

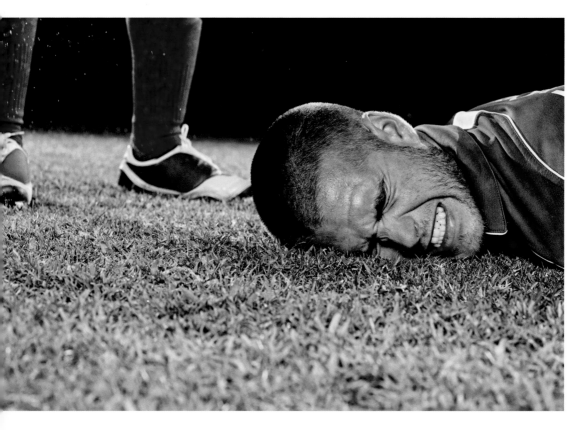

Vision must be regularly assessed by an ophthalmologist.

SPONTANEOUS INTRACRANIAL HYPOTENSION

This syndrome has been the subject of much recent research, and is now better understood. The symptoms can appear rapidly, and sometimes violently. The headache is diffuse and especially painful when the person is sitting or standing. The pain almost disappears when the person is lying down. If the disorder is severe, the person can only remain standing for a few minutes. In some cases, there may be nausea, tinnitus, and even double vision. Sometimes the pain radiates to the neck and shoulders, as if there were tension or downward traction starting at the nape of the neck. This headache is caused by a decrease in pressure in the head. The brain is surrounded by what is called the cerebrospinal fluid, or CSF. This fluid is contained in a membrane formed by the meninges, which envelop the brain and extend down into the spine to surround the spinal cord. It's possible for the membrane to be torn, whether by a small bony spur in the wrong place or perhaps following an accident. CSF leaks out through the hole, a bit like water in a sink when we pull out the plug. The pressure of CSF in the cranium then decreases, and when the person is standing, the brain tends to descend, pulling on the meninges and causing pain. The other symptoms are also explained by the downward displacement of the brain: traction on the auditory nerves causes tinnitus, and traction on the ocular nerves may result in double vision. In fact, spontaneous

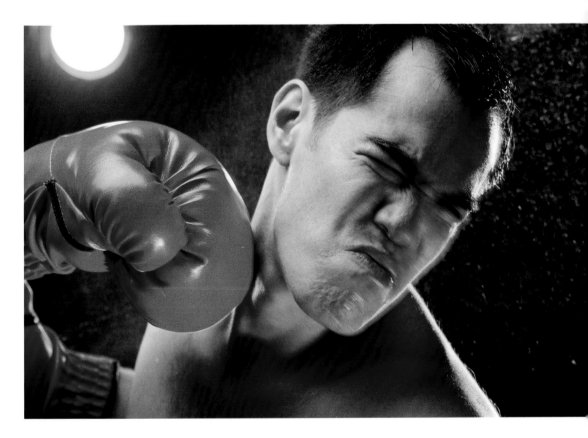

SPINAL TAP

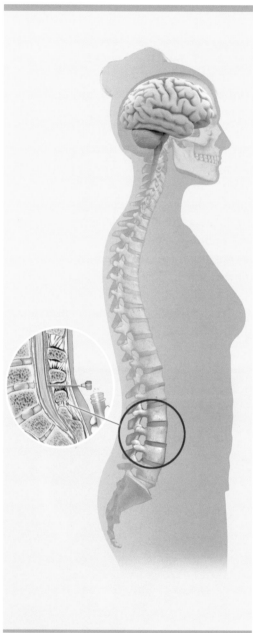

FIGURE 10

intracranial hypotension bears a strong resemblance to the kind of headache that may occur after a spinal tap or other needle-related procedures in the back (Figure 10). In these cases, the hole is caused by the procedure. The aim of treatment is to block the hole, usually using a technique called a blood patch, performed by an anaesthetist in a surgical unit. This kind of headache normally requires a neurological consultation.

NEW DAILY PERSISTENT HEADACHE (NDPH)

This type of headache remains a highly controversial topic. People with chronic headaches may receive this diagnosis when no specific cause is uncovered. The main characteristic of NDPH is the way it occurs. People usually describe a headache occurring on a specific day and even at a clearly defined time, whereas they never had headaches before. In some cases, a recent viral infection will be discovered, but no formal proof of an infectious cause has been established. The pain may resemble an ongoing migraine or a tension-type headache. It's interesting to note that the first series of patients suffering from this kind of headache, reported by a Canadian doctor in fact, described a spontaneous improvement a few months afterward. People diagnosed with NDPH, however, have often suffered from refractory headaches for years. Very often, how they occur is hard to specify, with sufferers not remembering the events very well. Recall bias is frequently observed, meaning that patients adapt their headache history to doctors' questions and they themselves end up adopting a very different version of remembered facts. In an NDPH situation, it's important to exclude other causes of chronic headache. There is no test for diagnosing NDPH, and no treatment has been specifically studied for this kind of headache. Most of the time, doctors will try the usual treatments for migraines.

Anyone with chronic disabling headaches should see a neurologist.

Headache is one of the most complex symptoms to explain and study. The correct diagnosis depends on a structured and attentive gathering of information about the patient's history, and imaging tests must only be asked for if a secondary cause is suspected. Migraine remains the most common diagnosis for a headache disorder.

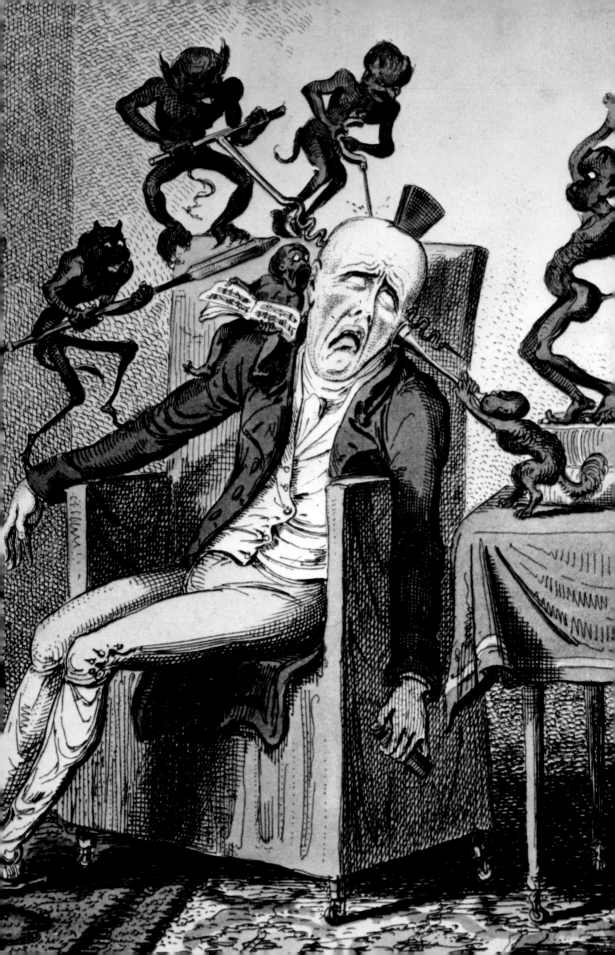

CHAPTER 2

The History of Migraine and Its Epidemiology

If you don't know history, then you don't know anything.
You are a leaf that doesn't know it is part of a tree.

— Michael Crichton

Migraine has afflicted human beings since the dawn of time. Reading ancient texts enables us to see how our understanding of this disease and its treatments has evolved (Figure 11). Migraine is still very widespread in modern society and has significant social and economic repercussions.

ANCIENT DESCRIPTIONS

When we read medical texts dating from Antiquity to the modern day, we realize that migraine symptoms have not changed very much over the centuries. It may be reassuring for some migraine sufferers to know that others before them have experienced the same symptoms.

EXPLANATORY THEORIES

The oldest explanations for migraines, as for most natural phenomena, made reference to gods and spirits. But, as is seen when the texts of the main pioneers are studied, the medical pendulum has always swung between various poles: the

↖ George Cruikshank, *Headache* (1819)

internal organs, the arteries, and the brain as an electrical organ. From Antiquity to the nineteenth century, there were two main theories based on observations about migraines: the theory of humours and the sympathetic theory. There were four humours: yellow bile, black bile, blood, and phlegm. These humours were used to explain many diseases and classify temperaments. Beginning with the first proposition of Galen (c.131–c.201), migraines were attributed to a yellow bile disorder, owing to the nausea and vomiting associated with the attacks. Migraine was believed to serve a purgative function. Other "secretory" symptoms, like diarrhea, excessive urination, sweating, and even tears, supported this theory. Even today, the term "feeling liverish" is sometimes used to describe migraines.

The word "sympathetic" as used by the Greeks had a completely different meaning than it does today. It meant an unconscious communication between the brain and the internal organs (see the Arab parchment on page 38). According to

ANCIENT DESCRIPTIONS

Period	Description
ANTIQUITY **HIPPOCRATES** (460–377 BCE) **AURA, NECK PAIN, RELIEF THROUGH VOMITING.**	As for Phoenix, this is more or less what he felt in his right eye: Most of the time he seemed to see something shining before him like a light, usually in part of the right eye. At the end of a moment, a violent pain supervened in the right temple, then in all the head and neck, and where the head is attached to the spine. Vomiting, when it became possible, was able to divert the pain and render it more moderate.
ANTIQUITY **ARETAEUS OF CAPPADOCIA** (30–90 CE) **NAUSEA, VOMITING, PHOTO- AND PHONOPHOBIA, DIZZINESS, FAINTING, IMPACT ON QUALITY OF LIFE.**	This is called heterocrania, an illness by no means mild, even though it intermits and although it appears to be slight. For if at any time it set in acutely […]; vertigo, deep-seated pain of the eyes as far as the meninges; irrestrainable sweat; sudden pain of the tendons, as of one striking with a club; nausea; vomiting of bilious matters; collapse of the patient.... For they flee the light; the darkness soothes their disease; nor can they bear readily to look upon or hear anything agreeable; their sense of smell is vitiated.... The patients, moreover, are weary of life, and wish to die.

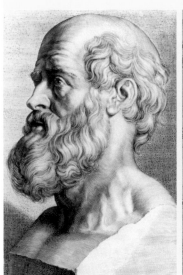

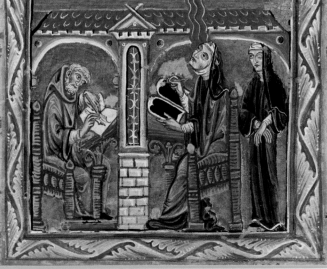

FIGURE 11   ↖ Hippocrates; Hildegard von Bingen

Period	Description
MIDDLE AGES HILDEGARD VON BINGEN (1098–1180) VISUAL AURA.	I saw a very large star, superb and magnificent, shooting southward accompanied by a multitude of falling stars…. Suddenly they were all annihilated, turned into pieces of coal, all black … and plunged into the abyss where they disappeared from my sight.
RENAISSANCE THOMAS WILLIS (1621–1675) CHRONIC MIGRAINE, FREQUENT AND LONG-LASTING ATTACKS, SLEEP DISORDERS, LONG-TERM PROGRESSION.	A few years ago, I was called to visit a very noble lady, ill for twenty years from an almost uninterrupted headache, which had at first been intermittent … she had been gravely afflicted by it…. This illness not being restricted to a single area of the head, it bothered her first on one side, then the other, and often everywhere in her head. During an attack (which almost always lasted more than a day and a night, and often lasted two, three, or four days), she could not tolerate light, talking, noise, or any movement; the room was kept dark, and she spoke to no one, did not sleep, and did not eat or drink anything. Afterward, toward the end of the attack, she used to lie down and sleep a deep and troubled sleep, from which she awoke in better condition…. Formerly, the attacks occurred only occasionally, and rarely on fewer than twenty days a month, but later, they occurred more frequently, and latterly, she was seldom free of them.
EDWARD LIVEING (1832–1919) ROLE OF GENETICS, IMPORTANCE OF THE NEUROLOGICAL SYSTEM, ATTACKS CAUSED BY INSTABILITY OF NERVOUS EQUILIBRIUM, CONCEPT OF THRESHOLD.	Explaining his theory of "nerve-storm," he described migraine and other "neuroses" in this way: … a certain tendency of the nervous system, for the most part innate and often hereditary, to the irregular accumulation and discharge of nerve-force …, a gradually increasing instability of equilibrium in the "nervous parts"; when this reaches a certain point, the balance of forces is liable to be upset and the train of paroxysmal phenomena determined by causes in themselves totally inadequate to produce such effects; just as a mere scratch will shiver to dust a mass of unannealed glass….

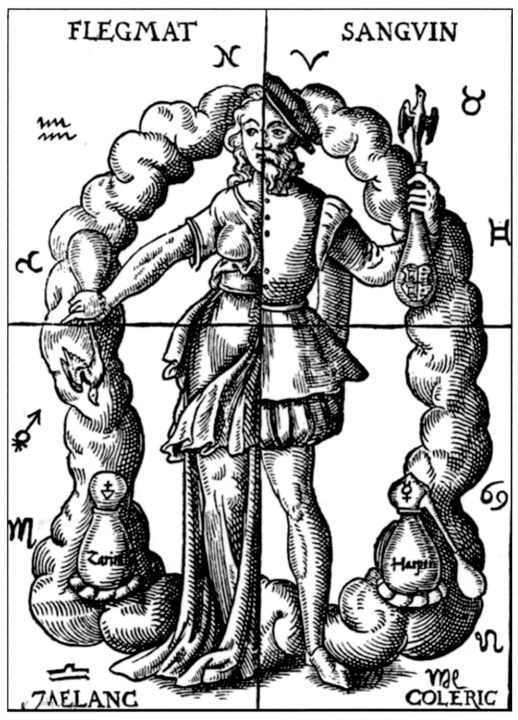

↗ The theory of humours (Hippocrates).The link between the brain and the digestive system.

this theory, intestinal or uterine blockages (constipation, menstruation) could trigger a migraine attack.

As Oliver Sacks emphasized in his book *Migraine*, these two theories were based on intimate communication between body and mind, between the internal organs and the brain. The nineteenth century saw the beginning of the development of the neurological sciences, and the focus shifted more specifically to the brain. At that time, our understanding of the neurological system, barely in its infancy, was still limited by the observation tools available, and psychiatry and neurology were closely related. This was the era of psychosomatic medicine and psychoanalysis. Remember that Freud himself had migraines. The origin of migraines was sought in the twists and turns of the psyche, in internal conflicts, hidden neuroses, or childhood traumas. The ancient purgative theories were adapted — instead of purging the organs, internal conflicts were "expelled." All migraines had to have a psychological cause. In the 1950s, science did not have access to the research techniques that will be described in Chapter 3. Brain function was hard to study, which gave free rein, in the world of migraines, to a set of psychoanalytical theories. These hypotheses may make us smile today, but they definitely caused harm to many migraine sufferers, who, in a way, were made to feel responsible for their symptoms.

In the 1970s, the psychoanalytic theory gave way to the vascular theory. The role of arterial pulsation in migraine headaches had already been recognized in Antiquity. Some migraineurs were described as having a sanguine temperament, with red migraines and crimson faces, as opposed

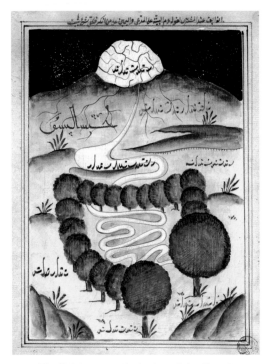

↗ The link between the brain and the digestive system.

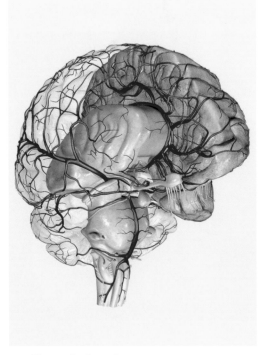

↗ The cerebral arteries.

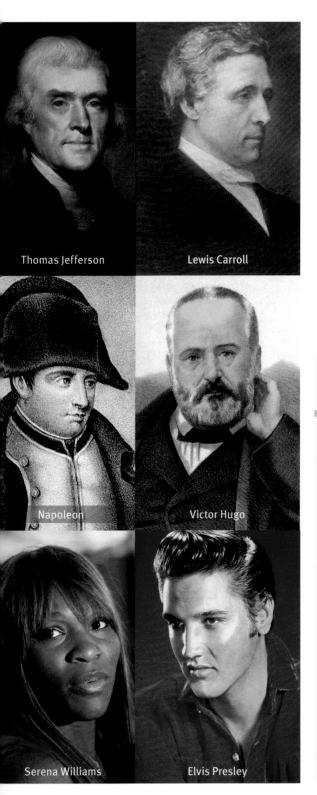

Thomas Jefferson

Lewis Carroll

Napoleon

Victor Hugo

Serena Williams

Elvis Presley

↗ A few famous migraineurs.

to white migraines, during which the face became deathly pale. English doctor Thomas Willis (1621–1675) had also proposed a theory based on spasms originating in the arteries and travelling along the nerves to the brain. According to this theory, reinforced by the observations of Harold Wolff (1898–1962), the dilation of the arteries in the head caused headaches, and the treatments used, like ergotamine, aimed to correct this dilation. Psychosomatic hypotheses were thus set aside, and migraine began to be considered an arterial problem, which meant that migraineurs, at least to some extent, no longer had to wear a psychiatric label.

Since the 1980s, with the advent of modern investigative techniques and

Psychoanalytic Interpretations

Furmanski (1952) wrote that nausea and vomiting were cardinal symptoms of migraine: they signified disgust and, in some cases of psychogenic vomiting, could be interpreted as the symbolic expulsion of a hated or feared situation or person.

Mansour (1957) claimed that migraine was a psychosomatic disease in which emotional factors played an important role. Attention focused quickly on the significance of periods of sexual frustration as migraine triggers. Some researchers described migraine sufferers as having obsessive-compulsive personality characteristics and difficulty managing generalized anger. Guilt made them repress this anger, which was later released during a migraine attack.

the development of molecular observation tools, attention has shifted to brain biochemistry and electrophysiology. Migraine is now viewed as a disorder of the central nervous system, of neurons themselves, and vascular problems are now considered to be the result rather than the cause. We will discuss these mechanisms, which summarize our current understanding of migraines, in the next chapter. Even though we can't help but be glad of scientific advances, the separation of body and mind, and even of the body into different organs studied separately, has occurred to the detriment of the big picture and a holistic view of the individual.

FAMOUS MIGRAINEURS

Since one person in ten suffers from migraines, it's not surprising to find many celebrities have had them. Migraineurs are found in the fields of literature, music, sport, and politics. This may be a source of encouragement and an example of perseverance for less famous migraineurs: being a migraine sufferer doesn't necessarily mean you can't reach your full potential. In the same way, the many descriptions of a migraine attack by famous writers, diplomats, and artists clearly prove that migraine spares no one and that the symptoms experienced, even though they vary, are quite similar overall.

THE TREATMENTS OF YESTERYEAR

When we consider treatments used in the past, it becomes obvious that the migraine sufferers of Antiquity must have been just as incapacitated by their attacks as migraineurs in the twenty-first century. Several of these treatments are still used today, in a modernized version. But it must be remembered that the length of time a treatment has been in use is no guarantee of its effectiveness. Difficulties with regard to the many migraine treatments whose effectiveness has been little demonstrated will be discussed in Chapter 5.

The oldest records of treatments for migraines have been found in Mesopotamia and date from nearly 4000 BCE. Later, like many other physicians in Antiquity, Aretaeus of Cappadocia (in the first century of our era) used bleeding. Since migraine is often accompanied by a pulsating sensation and a feeling of fullness in the head, draining a bit of blood may have seemed very logical to relieve an attack. Obviously, repeated bleedings could cause severe anemia. In spite of everything, these treatments certainly enjoyed lasting popularity; in the eighteenth century, Scottish physician Robert Whytt (1714–1766) was still using them. Dutch physician Pieter van Foreest (1521–1597), known as Forestus, was in the habit of prescribing the use of leeches, according to the same theory. The use of cupping glasses was another technique recommended by Hippocrates, Aretaeus, and Nicolaes Tulp, a seventeenth-century Dutchman. Cupping glasses are still recommended by some therapists, despite a lack of proof of their effectiveness.

A moderate treatment, recommended by Moses Maimonides (1135–1204), consisted of a hot bath, to "let the humours out," accompanied by a rose oil massage of the temples ... definitely a more pleasant treatment than being bled. The use of essential oils is still recommended for some patients, and there are studies on the use of menthol or peppermint oil. Many medicinal

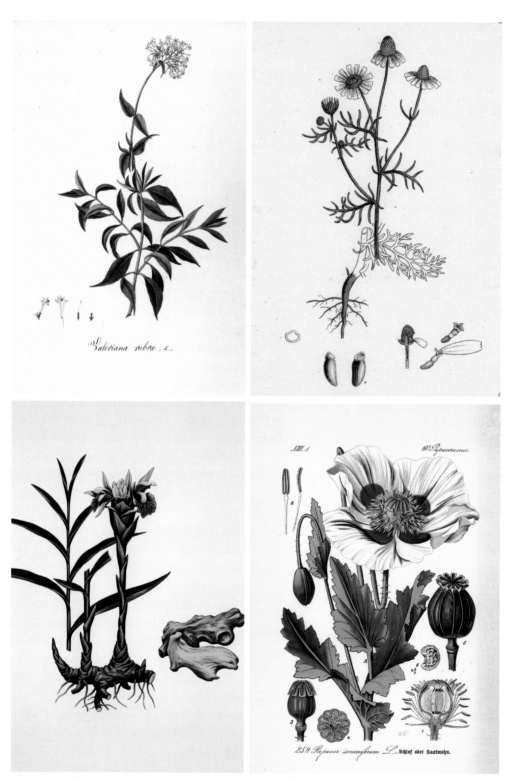

↗ Botanical treatments: valerian, camomile, ginger, opium (*papaver somniferum* poppy).

products have been used, including camomile, valerian, opium, and ginger.

Surgical treatments have also been tried. For refractory cases, Aretaeus proposed a more radical treatment: cauterization of the skull using a red-hot iron. To agree to this you had to be very desperate. This extreme technique was nonetheless used for centuries; Abulcasis, a physician at the court of the king of Spain in the tenth century, was still using it, but in a more complicated version. He recommended cutting the skin at the temples so as to insert a whole clove of garlic under the skin. We know that even in eighteenth-century France cauterization was still being used, as Claude Pouteau, a doctor from Lyon, commented on its use. The most extreme treatment was, without a doubt, trepanning — piercing a hole in the skull to "let the pressure out." While trepanning had likely been used since prehistoric times for other kinds of headaches, such as those caused by intracranial bleeding, it's probable that some migraineurs underwent this treatment.

We can assume from reading ancient texts that some patients must have been truly desperate to subject themselves to this kind of intervention. Nowadays, new surgical approaches are used. Many American clinics, for example, offer nerve decompression surgery that's supposed to cure migraines permanently. However, it's the opinion of the medical community that these operations are expensive and potentially dangerous, and no rigorous scientific study has proven their effectiveness.

Following the discovery of electricity, approaches based on this new knowledge were developed. Yet the Imperial Roman physicians Scribonius Largus (c.1–c.50) and Galen had already used electric rays to treat gout and headaches. In the nineteenth century, the neurosciences progressed rapidly. It was discovered that the arteries in the brain become wider or narrower (vasodilation or vasoconstriction) depending on nerve impulses from the sympathetic and parasympathetic systems. Obviously, this new way of interpreting migraine attacks was grist to the mill of electrotherapy. The arteries in the brain could now be stimulated electrically to keep them from dilating. Many scientists of the era tried using electrical stimulation, by means of a hydroelectric bath, for example.

The neurostimulation approach is still popular today, with several techniques under study, such as occipital or supraorbital

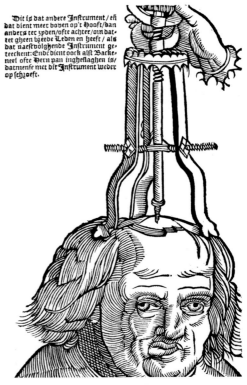

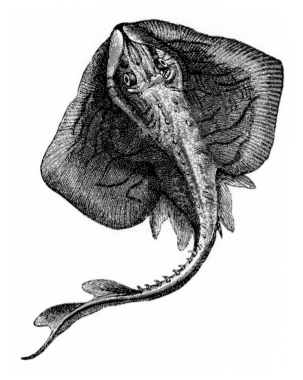

neurostimulation, transcranial magnetic stimulation, and non-invasive vagus nerve stimulation. In some cases, the electrical device has to be implanted, but other techniques use portable devices. Some patients also try techniques based on acupuncture, such as ear stapling. Doctors tend to be skeptical of this approach. All treatments must be studied scientifically before opinions based on solid information can be expressed.

MIGRAINE AND SOCIETY

Migraineurs often talk about their feelings of being alone and misunderstood by those around them. Yet migraine affects more than 10 to 12 percent of the population and almost 15 to 20 percent of women in their reproductive years! According to scientific studies, migraineurs have no reason to feel alone. On the contrary, given their numbers, they could form powerful associations and contribute to progress in research and access to care.

THE THIRD MOST COMMON DISEASE IN THE WORLD

According to a major study whose results were published in the prestigious journal *The Lancet* in 2012, migraine is the third most common disease in the world, in all categories. This makes it more common than all other better-known and more thoroughly studied diseases, like epilepsy, asthma, diabetes, and heart disease.

PREVALENCE WORLDWIDE

The prevalence of a disease refers to the percentage of people with a given

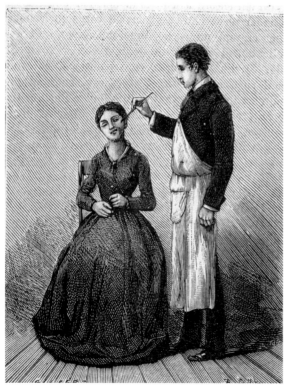

↗ From the electric ray to electrostimulation.

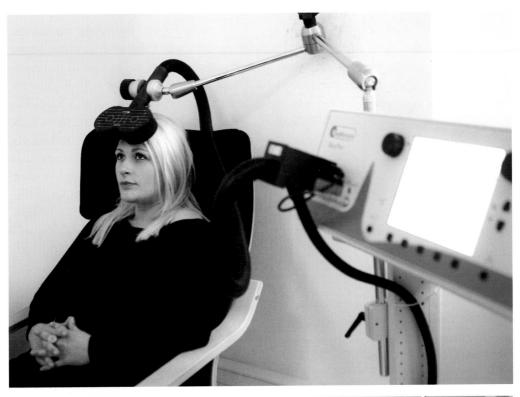

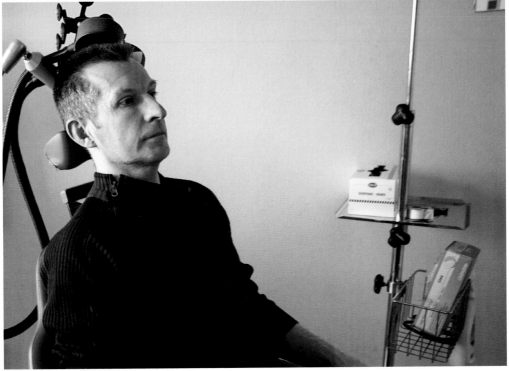

↗ Neurostimulation devices.

disease over a certain period of time in a sample of the population. The prevalence of migraine in adults, based on the most recent medical diagnostic criteria, has recently been reviewed (Figure 12). A fairly significant range has been observed: Italians have the highest prevalence of migraines at 21.7 percent, compared with Tanzanians, just 2.6 percent of whom suffer from migraines. Needless to say, epidemiological studies are not perfect. They can be distorted by flawed methodology, and the results must be interpreted with caution. An average prevalence of 10 to 12 percent has however been reported by numerous journals, based on a great many studies. One person in ten thus suffers from migraine, and nearly one woman out of every eight (Figure 13). What about children? Studies suggest an average prevalence of 7.7 percent. Before puberty, little boys are affected as much as little girls; at puberty, females begin to have migraines more than males do. In Canada, studies report a high prevalence: nearly 25 percent of women and 8 percent of men, for an average of 16.5 percent. According to a document prepared in 2010 by a consortium of Canadian experts, at least 1 percent of the Canadian population has more than five migraine attacks per month and from 1 to 2 percent have chronic migraine; this means that 3 percent of the population is affected by a

PREVALENCE OF MIGRAINE WORLDWIDE

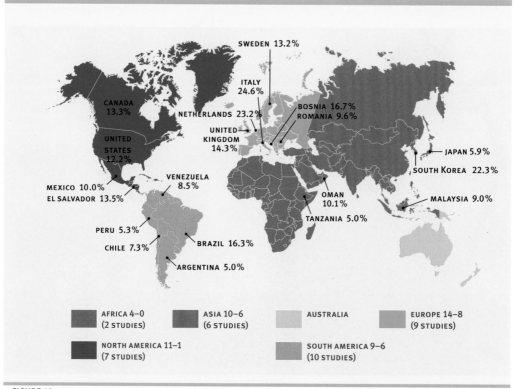

FIGURE 12

Adapted from L.J. Stovner et al., *Cephalalgia*, 2007.

severe form of migraine. Out of 35 million Canadians, this means that four million are migraine sufferers, with nearly one million having more than one attack a week.

THE FUNCTIONAL IMPACT OF MIGRAINE

A disease may be very common, like tooth decay, and not prevent people from functioning. If you have cavities, a few visits to the dentist will take care of them. But if you have migraine, the situation is different. Because it affects adults in the most productive years of their lives, migraine has significant repercussions on how those affected function on their personal, family, and professional lives.

Worldwide, migraines insidiously wreak havoc. Again according to the study

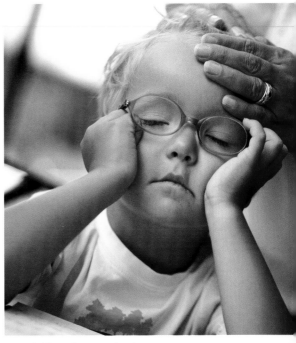

↗ Children also get migraines.

PREVALENCE OF MIGRAINE BY AGE AND SEX IN THE UNITED STATES

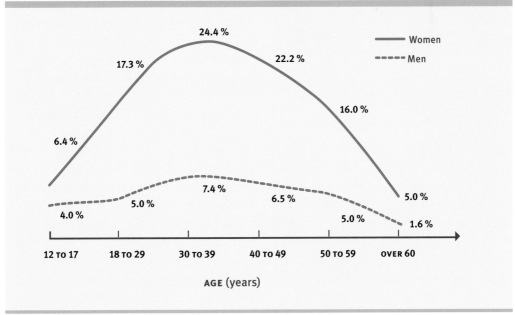

FIGURE 13

Adapted from R.B. Lipton, 2007.

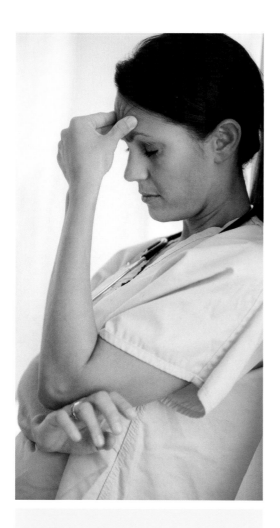

Migraine Is More Common in Neurologists!

Migraine affects 46 to 62 percent of neurologists, compared with 12 percent of the general population. Is it because they diagnose themselves more easily? Do they choose neurology because of their migraines? Whatever the reason, studies show that neurologists who are migraineurs know more about migraines, show greater empathy, and offer more attentive care.

published in *The Lancet* mentioned earlier, migraine is responsible for half the disability attributable to neurological disease (excluding vascular brain diseases). The criterion used, years lived with disability or YLDs, is calculated based on the frequency of the disease, in question, the number of years with the disease and the degree of disability during the symptomatic phases of the disease (Figure 14). Since migraine often begins at a young age and affects a large number of people, and since attacks prevent the individual from functioning, the result is impressive: migraine is the seventh-ranked cause of years lost because of disability, in all categories. Are you surprised? Are you skeptical? This is no doubt because we have a tendency to use individual cases to represent a disease. As a result, we have the impression that a brain tumour is much worse than migraine, since it can cause paralysis, epilepsy, and death. But brain tumours are very rare. When they aren't cured, the affected person dies as a result. The disability is thus concentrated in a fairly short period in a small number of people. Generally speaking, headaches have much higher social costs than most other neurological diseases (Figure 15).

It's estimated that seven million work days are lost annually because of migraine in Canada. According to a Canadian study done in 2005, each woman with migraines, on average, is unable to carry out her daily tasks for twenty-one days a year. Obviously, the more severe and frequent the attacks, the harder it is to function. Some people are completely unable to work while others miss one or two days a year.

WHY DOES MIGRAINE PREVENT FUNCTIONING?

Aside from days absent from work and spent in bed, days with reduced function must also be taken into account: the person manages to get to work, but cannot function normally. This is called presenteeism (as opposed to absenteeism). Migraineurs may spend the whole day staring at their computers, trying to concentrate on a meeting or a task, but, despite all their efforts, their ability to work is limited. There are several reasons for this: the migraine attack itself slows down cognitive function and is accompanied by difficulty in tolerating noises and light. The pain often increases

PROPORTION OF YEARS LIVED WITH DISABILITY (YLDS) CAUSED BY A NEUROLOGICAL DISEASE

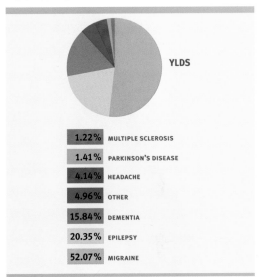

1.22%	MULTIPLE SCLEROSIS
1.41%	PARKINSON'S DISEASE
4.14%	HEADACHE
4.96%	OTHER
15.84%	DEMENTIA
20.35%	EPILEPSY
52.07%	MIGRAINE

FIGURE 14   Adapted from Vos, *The Lancet*, 2012.

COST OF DISORDERS OF THE BRAIN IN EUROPE

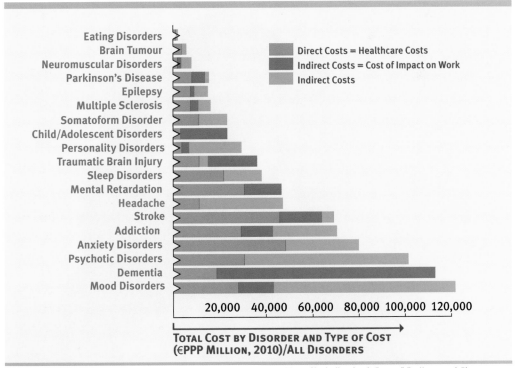

TOTAL COST BY DISORDER AND TYPE OF COST (€PPP MILLION, 2010)/ALL DISORDERS

FIGURE 15   Adapted from Gustavsson, "Cost of brain disorders in Europe," *Eur Neuropsych Pharm*, 2011.

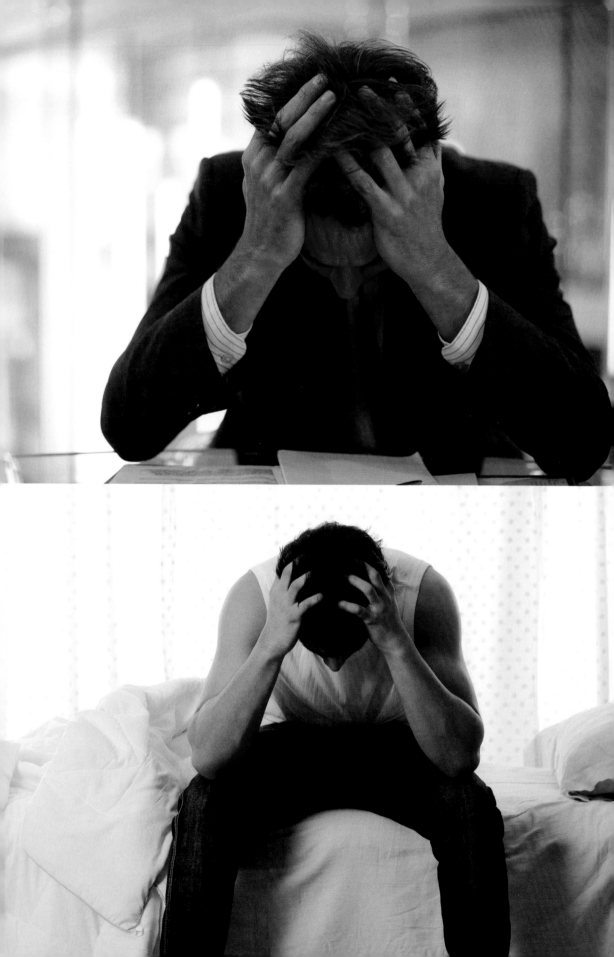

with physical or mental exertion. If the attack has been treated by taking a medication, the side effects of the treatment may also be felt, including fatigue, nausea, and difficulty concentrating. The hours and even the day after the attack is over often leave migraineurs in a weakened condition, "fragile, sensitive, exhausted." Fear that the attack will recur also leads people to curb their activities. The result: poorer performance at work or in personal activities ... and a great deal of guilt and low self-esteem. Outside the professional sphere, migraine also interferes with personal and social activities (Figure 16). Even when these are pleasant activities, migraine keeps you from functioning!

WHY IS MIGRAINE NOT TAKEN SERIOUSLY?

Migraine sufferers are often viewed with condescension by those around them. Certain expressions are so frequently reported that they've become classics in migraine clinics.

Given the avalanche of convincing data on the frequency of migraines and their socio-economic impact, we might expect that migraines would be a public health priority. But this is not at all the case. How can such a common and disabling disease be neglected in this way? In 2010, the Canadian Headache Society brought together a panel of experts to discuss how to improve care for migraines in Canada. They began by identifying the barriers limiting the quality of care (Figure 17). Among these, some of the characteristics of migraines no doubt explain part of the problem (Figures 18 A and B).

Annabel, 36

"My spouse doesn't understand why I have trouble functioning on the days I have a migraine, since I function normally every other day. At work, my employer looks at me with suspicion: did I really have a good reason to miss my meeting? As for my children, they've understood that when mummy is sick, they have to be quiet. Yet my doctor tells me over and over again that migraine is not really a serious problem and that my brain scan is normal. I don't know what to do.... How can I manage my life with all these migraines?"

MIGRAINE IS A COMPLEX NEUROLOGICAL DISEASE

It's fairly simple to explain that diabetes is caused by a lack of insulin, since the pancreas is destroyed. Similarly, Parkinson's disease is caused by a lack of dopamine, owing to the degeneration of the substantia nigra in the brain stem. Providing a simple overview of migraine, however, is quite a challenge. A migraine attack involves several different brain structures and neurotransmitters; this means that a curious person has to first understand something about neuroanatomy in order to grasp how the attack occurs. Migraine's complexity no doubt explains some of the prejudices associated with it. Since it can't be easily explained, the very existence of the disease is called into question.

IMPACT OF MIGRAINE ON PERSONAL LIFE

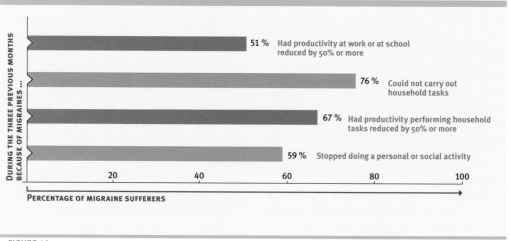

FIGURE 16

Adapted from Lipton, *Headache*, 2001.

BARRIERS TO OPTIMAL MIGRAINE MANAGEMENT

1   There is a significant stigma attached to a migraine diagnosis. Often considered to be a psychiatric disorder, migraine is often the subject of jokes in poor taste.

2   The repercussions of migraines on work are underestimated by employees and employers.

3   Acute migraine treatments are under-prescribed. If treated with non-prescription painkillers, patients become victims of medication-overuse headaches, a problem whose importance is underestimated.

4   Preventive treatments are underutilized. Many patients who should be treated are not.

5   Non-pharmacological approaches for migraine treatment are hard to find and not used enough.

FIGURE 17

Adapted from Becker,*CMAJ*, 2010, critères déterminés lors du Forum canadien sur la migraine, 2006.

MIGRAINE IS INVISIBLE

The neurological phenomena causing migraine are invisible on available clinical imaging examinations. A migraine attack is caused by inflammatory and electrical mechanisms that occur on a microscopic scale and leave no traces in the brain (or only very subtle traces) when the attack is over. This feature of migraine contributes to doubts about its existence: what we don't see, we don't believe in, especially nowadays, when tomography and magnetic resonance imaging are easily accessible.

RESTRAINTS ON PROACTIVITY

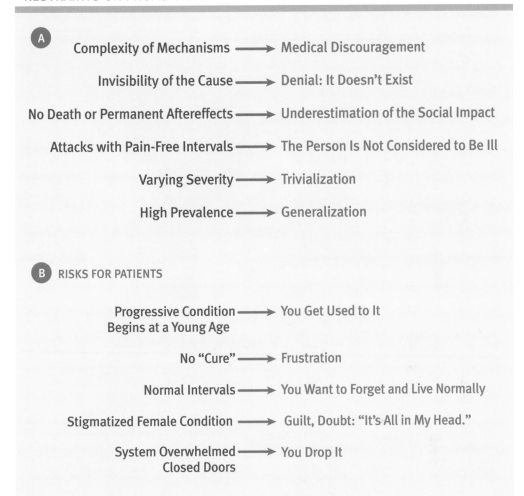

A

Complexity of Mechanisms	→	Medical Discouragement
Invisibility of the Cause	→	Denial: It Doesn't Exist
No Death or Permanent Aftereffects	→	Underestimation of the Social Impact
Attacks with Pain-Free Intervals	→	The Person Is Not Considered to Be Ill
Varying Severity	→	Trivialization
High Prevalence	→	Generalization

B RISKS FOR PATIENTS

Progressive Condition Begins at a Young Age	→	You Get Used to It
No "Cure"	→	Frustration
Normal Intervals	→	You Want to Forget and Live Normally
Stigmatized Female Condition	→	Guilt, Doubt: "It's All in My Head."
System Overwhelmed Closed Doors	→	You Drop It

FIGURE 18   Elizabeth Leroux.

MIGRAINE IS NOT A DEGENERATIVE DISEASE

Even though a migraineur's brain shows features visible in medical imaging, it continues to function ... most of the time. Migraine doesn't have an impact on mortality and doesn't cause visible handicaps, like paralysis or loss of language. This reality also influences people's perceptions: you don't die from migraine. Death remains, for human beings, the worst outcome. But what's the value of a life made difficult by chronic pain?

MIGRAINE IS A PAROXYSMAL DISEASE

This means it's characterized by attacks interspersed with normal periods during which the person can function. Migraine can be described according to the frequency of its attacks. This kind of pattern also contributes to prejudices about migraine:

53

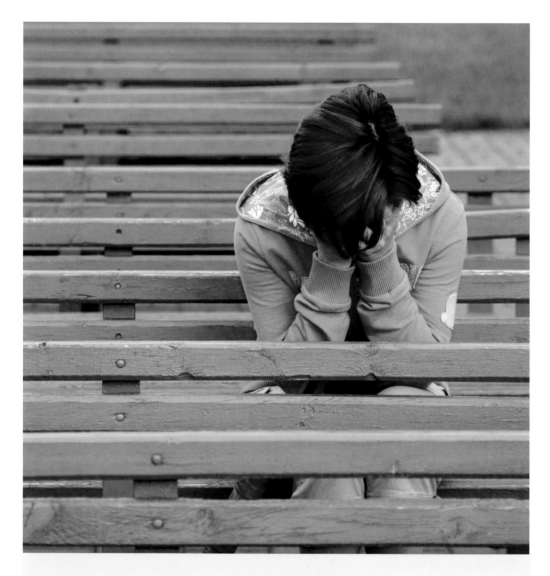

Ten Things Not to Say to a Migraine Sufferer

1. Sometimes I get headaches too.
2. Think about something else; things will get better.
3. You should stop ... eating chocolate, drinking alcohol, etc.
4. It's all in your head.
5. My best friend's aunt tried this treatment. You should try it!
6. At least it won't kill you.
7. In the end things will get better. You just have to be patient.
8. I'd really like to be able to stay home all the time like you.
9. It's just that you don't know how to manage stress.
10. Maybe it's your sinuses.

close friends and family, doctors, and employers, just to name a few, have great difficulty accepting that someone can be unable to function for a day and then go back to normal. In the case of chronic migraine, sometimes the brain never goes back to normal but remains constantly in a dysfunctional state. That also makes those close to the sufferer skeptical: it may seem impossible to them to have a constant headache.

MIGRAINE IS A DISEASE WHOSE SEVERITY VARIES

Compared with cystic fibrosis, heart disease, or muscular dystrophy, which almost invariably become progressively worse and involve significant disability, migraine affects a large portion of the population, but not with the same severity. A large percentage of migraine sufferers will never have frequent or severe attacks. This fact also influences our perception of migraine: so many people have migraine and don't complain! This makes it easy to cast doubt on those people with migraine who are in the group that experiences its most severe effects. Why does Mrs. Smith have to take three medications and sometimes go to emergency, while Mrs. Johnson, on the other hand, manages her attacks very well with Advil? Human beings' natural tendency to standardize makes life difficult for researchers and patients by trivializing the disease.

Migraine didn't start yesterday. It exists, it has been causing humanity pain for thousands of years, and it affects billions of people.

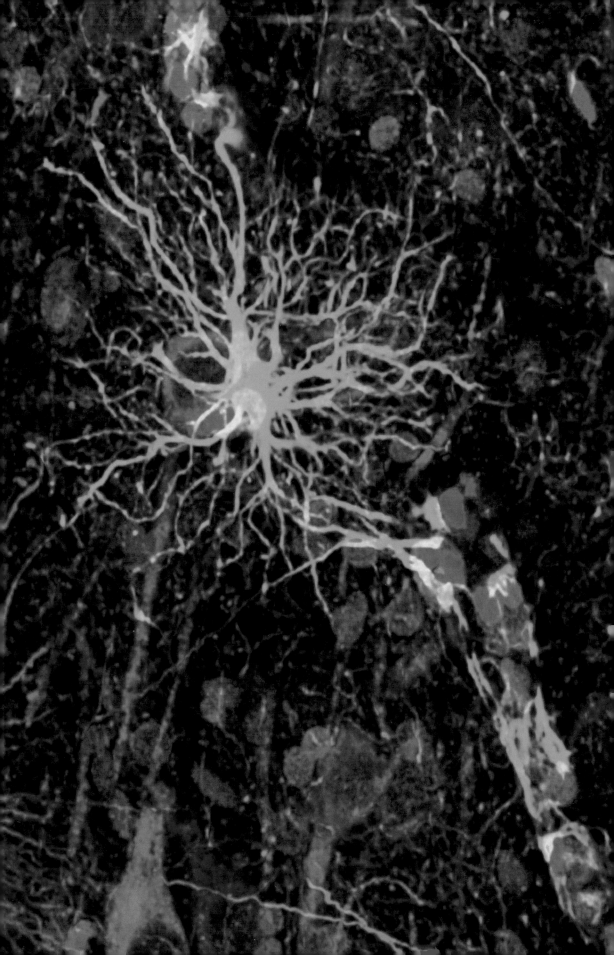

CHAPTER 3

Symptoms and Biology of a Migraine Attack

If you can't explain it simply,
you don't understand it well enough.

— ALBERT EINSTEIN

The brain is at the root of who we are, how we think, what we perceive and feel. It manages almost all of our biological functions. But here's the thing — the brain is not easy to analyse! Its functioning is much more complex than that of the other organs. It contains nearly 85 billion neurons that interact every second with other neurons organized in networks. These neurons communicate with each other using electrical and chemical mechanisms that can't be studied with the naked eye. It's therefore impossible to explain what happens during a migraine attack without first giving an overview of brain function.

The parable of the elephant and the blind men (see the following page) illustrates clearly how hard it is to acquire a coherent understanding of something when it can't be seen in its entirety. Migraine research uses several approaches, each providing new elements of knowledge, but none making it currently possible to summarize everything into a comprehensive framework. No scientist yet knows what initial event triggers a migraine attack, but, owing to the work of thousands of researchers, we now know what some of its stages are. Before describing these stages, it's important to describe a few brain structures.

RESEARCH TECHNIQUES

Several research techniques can be used to explore aspects of migraine (Figure 19). These techniques can be applied to animals as well as humans. Conventional tomodensitometry and magnetic resonance imaging are not very useful, however.

ELECTROPHYSIOLOGY
The brain's electrical activity can now be studied in animals using electrodes implanted in specific groups of neurons. This makes it possible, for example, to study how the electrical response of the trigeminal nucleus changes in reaction to different stimuli and certain medications.

↖ The migraine trio: neurons, arteries, astrocytes.

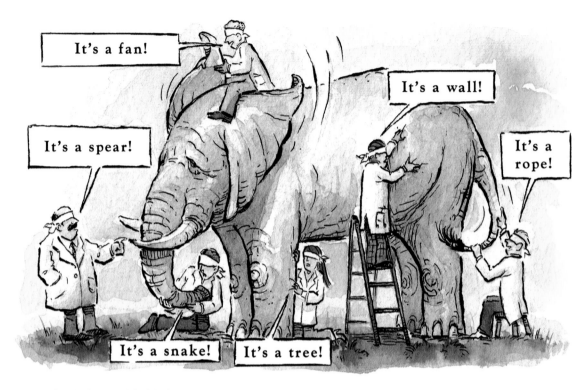

↗ The elephant and the blind men.

This technique cannot be used in humans, since it wouldn't be acceptable to implant electrodes in a living patient simply for research purposes. Electrical currents, called evoked potentials, observe the brain's response to an image, a sound, a touch. They can be recorded by surface electrodes. This technique, used in humans, allows us to see how the brain manages these stimuli, but with a limited degree of accuracy.

BIOLOGICAL ANALYSES

Using blood tests, the levels of various substances in the bloodstream during and between attacks can be measured. This can give an idea of what's going on in the brain, but this technique has limitations, as a number of non-brain factors can influence the levels of the different substances studied in the bloodstream. Blood tests are an integral part of pharmaceutical research, enabling us to understand fully the metabolism of a prescribed medication.

FUNCTIONAL IMAGING

By means of positron emission tomography (PET) scans and functional magnetic resonance imaging (fMRI), the activity of various brain regions in a variety of contexts can be observed. In general, the consumption of glucose is measured by assuming that the more active a neuron is, the more glucose it consumes. Observing the activity of a neuron using functional imaging doesn't allow us to say accurately what the effect of this activity is. For example, a group of very active neurons can stimulate or inhibit other neurons; the

RESEARCH TECHNIQUES

	Level of Observation	Structure or Mechanism Observed	Research Tools
	Macroscopic (visible to the naked eye)	Brain, meninges, arteries	Functional imaging: CT scan (tomodensitometry), MRI
	Electrical	Neuronal activity	Electrophysiological studies
	Chemical	Proteins Neurotransmitters Ionic channels	Blood tests Cellular markers Analysis of proteins
	Metabolic	Blood flow in various areas of the brain in real time	Functional MRI PET (positron emission tomography)
	Genetic	DNA, chromosomes	Genetic analyses

FIGURE 19   Elizabeth Leroux.

results must therefore be interpreted with caution. Using some of these imaging techniques, we can also study the metabolism of specific neurotransmitters, like serotonin or dopamine. The images generated by these techniques are not very accurate, but provide an idea of the active areas in a given situation.

GENETIC STUDIES
The activity of neurons, like that of all the other cells in the human body, is regulated by genes. Genes are what determines how a cell develops, becomes specialized, and interacts with its environment. Genetics is therefore the basis of all of the human body's functioning. It's

important to stress that all the networks in the body are influenced by hundreds, or even thousands of genes, and that while some diseases are caused by a single gene (monogenic), others are determined by hundreds or thousands of interdependent genes (polygenic). This makes it very difficult to find *the* gene responsible for a particular problem. Genetic studies can be carried out by means of chromosome analysis or by observing the transmission of a disease in families, twins, or ethnic groups.

AT THE MACROSCOPIC LEVEL: BRAIN STRUCTURES

The brain is made up of several distinct structures that interact with each other. To better understand migraine attacks, the brain's anatomy first has to be described (Figure 21), and a few concepts about neuronal function presented.

THE CORTEX
The cortex is composed of neurons, the brain's electrical cells. The cortex is the outer layer of neurons that communicate with each other. It's divided into lobes, each with its own function, such as motor skills, vision, or language. These electrical cells in the brain function in a binary way: they either discharge or they don't, somewhat like a switch that's either on or off. Neurons communicate with each other by means of electrical signals and neurotransmitters.

THE MENINGES
The meninges surround and protect the brain. They are very sensitive to pain and

inflammation. This is why meningitis produces very intense headaches.

THE ARTERIES
The arteries are essential for the brain, as they carry the oxygen and nutrients required for neurons to function. They are very sensitive to pain, containing nerve fibres that can sense various stimuli, like inflammation, for example.

THE NERVES
A nerve is sort of like an electrical cable. A neuron sends a message, which a nerve then transmits from a distance using electrical current. Nerve endings have receptors sensitive to various stimuli: chemical, thermic, mechanical. Each stimulus can be translated into an electrical signal that travels toward the body of the neuron, which then uses this information to communicate with other neurons. There are twelve cranial nerves that ensure the functioning of the organs in the head — smell, vision, hearing, taste, movements of the face and mouth, as well as the secretion of tears and saliva. The fifth cranial nerve is very important for our understanding of migraine, as it transmits sensations from the head. Since it has three main branches, it's known as the trigeminal nerve. This is the nerve that transmits sensations from the face, teeth, and sinuses, but also from the arteries inside the skull and the meninges. The brain itself is completely insensitive to pain, as it isn't innervated by sensory nerve endings.

THE BRAIN STEM AND THE NUCLEI
The brain stem, so called because all the nerves branch off from it, is a major centre in the brain. It contains the nuclei, which

PHASES OF A MIGRAINE ATTACK

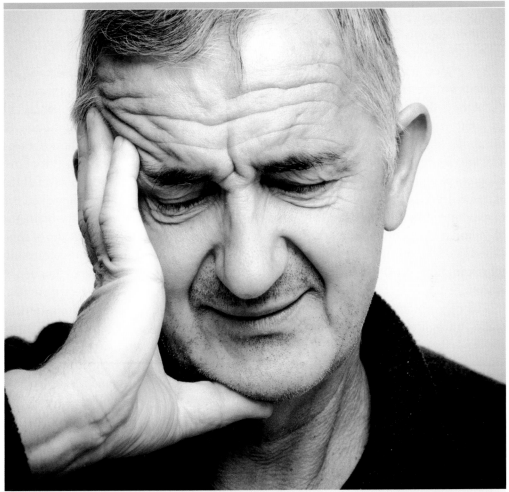

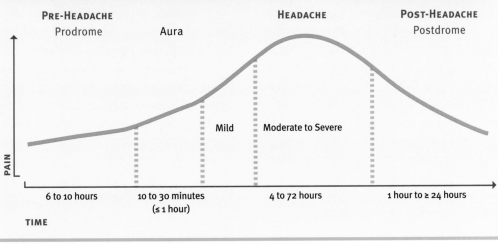

FIGURE 20

are in fact clumps of specialized neurons grouped together to perform a specific function, like sensation, motor skills, and secretion. Several nuclei are important in a migraine attack. The median raphe nucleus synthesizes the serotonin found throughout the brain. The periaqueductal gray matter modulates painful sensations, somewhat like a dimmer on a light fixture. This area is very powerful. It's even able to suppress pain sensations, in situations of extreme stress, for example. It's important to remember that the brain is always able to modulate pain intensity via what are called the descending control pathways, which include the periaqueductal gray matter.

The trigeminal nucleus receives information transmitted by the trigeminal nerve and sends it to the thalamus.

THE THALAMUS AND THE HYPOTHALAMUS

The thalamus is like a miniature brain. It's a relay point, an exchange area for all of the brain's activities, except the sense of smell. This means that everything entering or leaving the brain goes through the thalamus. It could be described as a large integrator. The thalamus also contains several nuclei responsible for communication between the brain stem and the cortex. The hypothalamus controls the pituitary gland and thus the endocrine system. It's a very tiny, but extremely important, structure. The body's functioning depends on it to regulate hunger, thirst, sleep, and the stress response. The hypothalamus receives, among other things, information on light perceived by the eyes to synchronize the wake-sleep cycle.

AT THE MICROSCOPIC LEVEL: ELECTRICITY AND CHEMICAL COMMUNICATION

The structures we've just described are visible using imaging techniques such as tomography and magnetic resonance, but they appear normal in migraineurs. To fully understand migraine attacks, we also have to describe how these structures function at a microscopic level, the level of the cell, which is not visible to the naked eye (Figure 22). The main cells of the brain, the neurons, have two principal modes of communication: electricity and neurotransmitters. Sometimes the two systems function in sequence; for example, an electrical signal will trigger the release of neurotransmitters. A single neuron constantly receives information from thousands of others. The result: electrical activity that varies in intensity and speed, and the synthesis and release of neurotransmitters to a greater or lesser degree. The release of certain neurotransmitters may cause the arteries to dilate or narrow, depending on the neuron's needs. In the case of a migraine attack, the release of neurotransmitters results in neurogenic inflammation.

As a result, to study migraine, we need the ability to observe the electrical activity of neurons and their chemical exchanges. This is however much more difficult than capturing a static image of the brain at a precise moment! New techniques have been developed by scientists and will no doubt lead to a better understanding of migraine attacks.

STAGES OF A MIGRAINE ATTACK

Migraine is much more than a headache. In fact, migraine attacks are really constellations of symptoms in sequences that vary from one individual to another. The classic sequence of these stages consists of prodrome, aura, headache, and postdrome (Figure 20). Each stage is the subject of research, and to explain migraine attacks it's simpler to present them separately, by describing for each the underlying mechanisms currently understood (Figure 23).

THE ONSET OF THE ATTACK: THE THRESHOLD PRINCIPLE

What causes the brain stem to trigger inflammation is still not precisely known, but there are many theories on the table. First of all, a migraine attack may occur in response to an imbalance in the brain that triggers an aura in the cortex (an electrical wave) or prodrome in the hypothalamus. The onset of this kind of attack might therefore be related to an imbalance in brain metabolism: strong emotion, fluctuation in estrogen levels, alcohol consumption, coffee withdrawal, etc.

Second, the inflammation might be triggered by external nerve irritation: the face, sinuses, eyes, neck — all of these sensitive structures can influence the trigeminal nerve and trigger the attack cascade.

In both cases, a threshold must be reached for the attack to be triggered.

These two kinds of triggers have a direct effect on treatments. It's possible to reduce imbalances in brain function and alleviate potentially irritating external sensations. It's also possible to limit the brain's sensitivity to these imbalances and stimuli or, in other words, to raise the trigger threshold for attacks.

THE PRODROME, A PREPARATORY PHASE?

In the twelve hours before a crisis, 30 percent of migraine sufferers report premonitory symptoms. The most common are fatigue, mood swings, gastrointestinal upsets, and neck pain. They also mention yawning, more frequent urination, mild nausea, and photophobia. All of these symptoms could be caused by abnormal activation of the hypothalamus. The prodrome can last less than one hour to ten hours.

AURA, OR THE RESULT OF AN ELECTRICAL WAVE

Almost 30 percent of migraine sufferers experience auras, whose frequency varies greatly. Auras often appear as visual symptoms that occur gradually. Patients report many "visions" consisting of bright and sometimes colourful dots, flashes, kaleidoscopes, and complex shapes. Other more subtle descriptions include blurred, greyish vision, as if the person were looking through a heat wave. The figures on page 66 are drawings provided by patients, showing the wide variety of visual auras. This variety is made possible by the great complexity of the visual cortex. In some cases, auras are sensory or phasic; in other words, patients report gradually increasing numbness on one side of the body or difficulties in speaking, reading, or understanding what people say to them. In more severe cases and in genetic forms of migraine, aura may even lead to paralysis on one side of the body, coma, and fever. These forms, however, are extremely rare, and doctors must then carry out an extensive examination to exclude all the other medical conditions that might cause these symptoms.

Aura symptoms can now be explained by the discovery of cortical spreading depression (CSD). This is an electrical wave that travels from neuron to neuron across the cortex and produces symptoms specific to

MACROSCOPIC: BRAIN ANATOMY

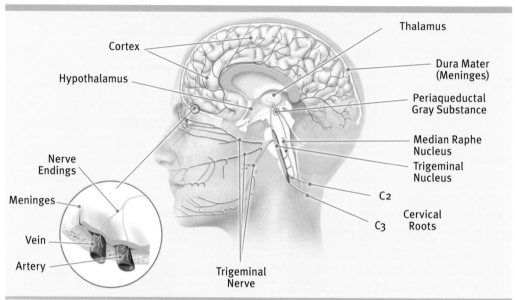

FIGURE 21

MICROSCOPIC: AT THE CELLULAR LEVEL

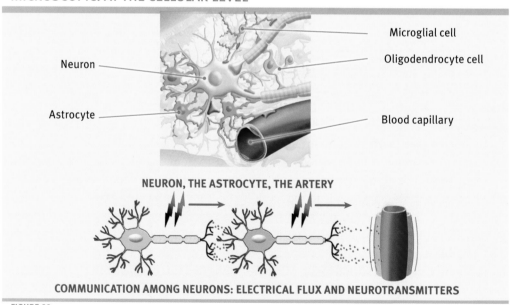

FIGURE 22

STAGES OF A MIGRAINE ATTACK

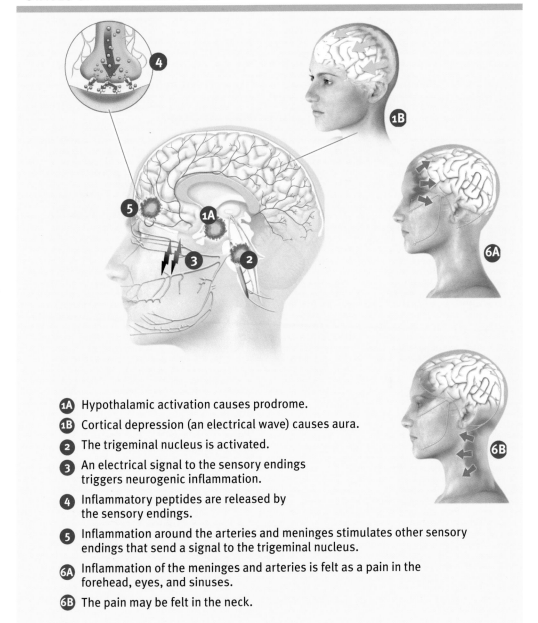

1A Hypothalamic activation causes prodrome.

1B Cortical depression (an electrical wave) causes aura.

2 The trigeminal nucleus is activated.

3 An electrical signal to the sensory endings triggers neurogenic inflammation.

4 Inflammatory peptides are released by the sensory endings.

5 Inflammation around the arteries and meninges stimulates other sensory endings that send a signal to the trigeminal nucleus.

6A Inflammation of the meninges and arteries is felt as a pain in the forehead, eyes, and sinuses.

6B The pain may be felt in the neck.

FIGURE 23

the area involved. An attack on the occipital lobe will produce visual symptoms; on the parietal lobe, sensory symptoms, like numbness, etc. This wave can be studied in the laboratory, but only on animals. CSD may be compared to an electrical and chemical storm that seriously disturbs neuronal function. In cases where patients report dots of light followed by loss of vision, it's thought that the light-related symptoms are caused by neuronal discharge, while vision loss results from a temporary halt in neuronal activity.

We now know that aura might trigger a headache by acting on the trigeminal nucleus from a distance, since the two structures are connected. Studies on animals have shown that when CSD occurs it can activate the trigeminal nucleus and thus trigger a migraine attack. This is why most patients report that their symptoms appear before the headache. Generally speaking, however, auras do not seem to be the cause of migraines, since most patients don't experience them. Furthermore, many patients, when specifically asked, say that when aura begins the headache has already started, even if it's mild. It's

therefore also possible for activation in the trigeminal nucleus to trigger an aura. In many cases, the connections between brain structures function in both directions.

HEADACHE, PAIN

Migraine pain is a little like a burn that's triggered all by itself in the brain and is felt in the face and neck. To explain this phenomenon clearly, we have to take the time to present two concepts: neurogenic inflammation (produced by the brain) and referred pain (remote pain).

THE CAUSE OF THE PAIN: NEUROGENIC INFLAMMATION

Migraine pain results from inflammation inside the cranium. If you're wondering what inflammation is, think back to your last sunburn. The four signs of inflammation are redness, heat, swelling, and pain. Note that the first three signs are directly related to vasodilation, which allows blood flow to the inflamed area to increase. Inflammation is usually triggered by a disruption in the organism (infection, injury) requiring immune system intervention and tissue repair.

The brain stem is responsible for migraine inflammation. In response to a trigger, the trigeminal nucleus is activated. It sends an electrical message to the fibres surrounding the brain arteries and meninges (very sensitive structures) and releases peptides, which are inflammatory substances. Imagine the following situation: your brain decides to sprinkle ground cayenne pepper on your meninges! This irritates the nerve fibres and sends a painful signal back to the brain stem. The trigeminal nucleus then passes on the information to the thalamus, which sends it to

↖ Auras drawn by patients (L.P. Queiroz et al., *Cephalalgia*, 2011)

the cortex, where it's interpreted as pain. This very important and complex process is called neurogenic inflammation. The term means that the inflammation is caused by a brain process and not by injury. There are many inflammatory substances involved in a migraine attack, but one is of particular interest to us: CGRP (calcitonin gene-related peptide). This highly irritating substance is a prime therapeutic target.

THE LOCATION OF THE PAIN: REFERRED PAIN

Neurogenic inflammation originates in the brain. However, most migraineurs experience pain in the forehead, eyes, temples, and even the sinuses. This can be explained by the principle of referred pain.

The best known example of this is the pain in the left arm during a myocardial infarction, or heart attack. The brain incorrectly interprets pain coming from the heart, which is lacking oxygen, whereas the left arm is not at all injured.

Our brain contains a geographical map of our skin. It's perfectly able to distinguish between pressure on a toe and pressure on a finger. Similarly, the face is precisely innervated. A single eyelash falling on the cheek is quickly detected by branches of the trigeminal nerve. However, our body's internal organs are not represented quite so clearly. For example, we are not aware (fortunately) of each centimetre of our colon! Inside the cranium, the arteries, veins, and meninges can be painful, but the brain doesn't have a detailed "geographical" sensory map of our meninges and our arteries. Pain stemming from these structures is therefore hard to locate or is perceived as coming from other, better represented, areas, like the face and neck.

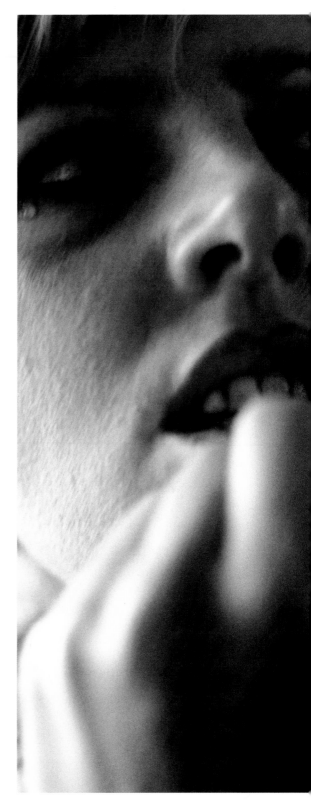

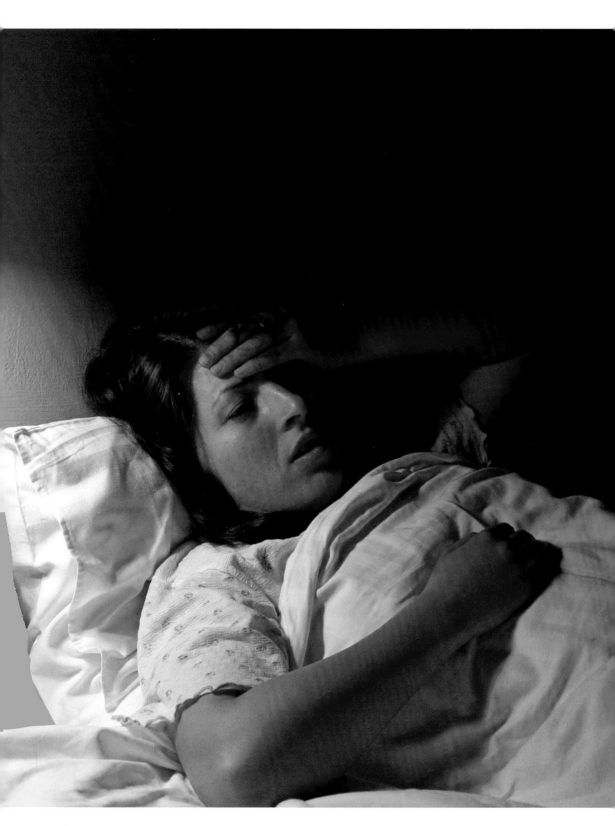

A very large number of migraineurs blame their migraines on neck problems. Several studies have shown that migraine attacks are accompanied by neck pain in almost 70 percent of patients, even in the absence of neck injuries or persistent neck pain between attacks. Neck pain can also occur in the prodrome stage. To fully understand this, we have to return to the concept of referred pain. The neck is innervated by cervical nerve roots (C2 and C3), which also affect an area of the skin on the back of the skull and on the neck (Figure 21). These roots are also connected to the central trigeminal nucleus, which receives all the information coming from the head and face. This anatomical convergence is the source of head-neck referred pain.

PAIN PULSATILITY

Pain pulsatility is one of the diagnostic criteria for migraine. From Antiquity onward, this pulsatility was attributed to the arterial pulse. Very often, patients are asked if they feel a throbbing pain, like a "pulse in the head." Imagine the surprise of American researchers when, after asking migraine sufferers during an attack to beat the rhythm of the painful pulsation, they realized that this rhythm was completely different from the subjects' heartbeats! Through a very simple experiment, they had just challenged a theory that went back more than two thousand years — that migraine pain was a mere reflection of arterial hypersensitivity.

ALLODYNIA AND SENSITIZATION

Allodynia is a word that means "everything hurts." For example, an allodynic area on the skin will feel pain from slight cold or heat and even from a gentle touch. Allodynia is caused by a change in sensory

Claudia, 32

Claudia gets frequent migraine headaches, often lasting three full days, and the attacks are very difficult to manage, even with prescriptions from her doctor. On the second day of the attack, she begins to be very sensitive to touch. She can no longer stand wearing her glasses. She can no longer tie her hair back. Even the feel of a pillow against her face is unpleasant, especially on the right side, which is the most painful. Her neck gets stiff and her partner, who gives her a massage to relax her, realizes that the pressure on her shoulders is more painful than soothing. At this point in the attack, Claudia knows that no treatment will work. Worst of all is the feeling that she's crazy. How can normal sensations hurt so much?

neuron function called sensitization. The perception thresholds are lowered and the neurons react to weaker stimuli that they shouldn't even transmit in normal conditions. They may even begin to perceive sensations outside their usual perception range. Think back to your last burn: hot water feels like its boiling, touch becomes painful, and you can feel your pulse in the tip of your finger. The chain of transmission between the skin and the cortex includes three groups of neurons (skin–spinal cord, spinal cord–thalamus, thalamus–cortex), and sensitization may occur at each level. It can be triggered by nerve damage, or by repeated painful stimuli. It's thought that a combination of neurogenic inflammation and sensitization is at play when migraines become more frequent or chronic.

PHOTOPHOBIA, OR DIFFICULTY TOLERATING LIGHT

"During a migraine, the only thing I can do is lie down in a dark room...." Light is often hard for migraine sufferers to tolerate. During an attack, 80 percent of patients describe this kind of photophobia, in varying degrees. In chronic migraineurs, this problem may persist even between attacks. But where does this light-related "pain" come from? Most of the time, light is associated instead with happy feelings, a beautiful spring morning, summer holidays, etc.

There are two types of photophobia. On one hand, light may make the headache more intense. On the other, light may be perceived more intensely, even unpleasantly. The origin of these two types of photophobia lies in the anatomical pathways connecting the retina to the thalamus and to the trigeminal nucleus. Interestingly, migraineurs who've gone blind owing to degeneration of the retina can nonetheless experience photophobia if their receptors specific to the thalamus have been preserved. Migraine sufferers are also very sensitive to sounds (sonophobia or phonophobia) and to smells (osmophobia), but these symptoms are not as well understood as photophobia.

NAUSEA AND VOMITING

Nausea and vomiting are caused by a structure in the brain stem called the area postrema. Obviously, this structure receives information from many systems, including those for balance, digestion, and pain. It's also very sensitive to a wide range of substances (including drugs) and may be sensitive to the strong emotions analyzed in the limbic lobe as well. Similarly, intestinal function is influenced by the brain stem and the sympathetic system. This makes it likely (but for the time being undemonstrated) that a migraine attack's electrical storm involves the areas that control the digestive system, causing symptoms of nausea, vomiting, and sometimes diarrhea. Some patients notice that vomiting alleviates the attack and may even end it, but this process is still poorly understood.

DIZZINESS

Migraine is associated with a great many disorders of the balance system (called the vestibular system), such as Ménière's disease and motion sickness. Although dizziness and vertigo are not diagnostic criteria for migraine, they are reported by some patients. When vertigo is frequently experienced during a migraine attack, in the absence of any other disease, the term vestibular migraine is used. The exact cause of this relationship is not yet known.

THE END OF THE ATTACK AND POSTDROME

Even without any treatment, a migraine attack ends naturally in most patients. The mechanisms that interrupt migraine attacks are still unknown. During the hours and sometimes days that follow an attack, it's not uncommon to feel great fatigue or perhaps a very slight headache. In other people, when the attack has been treated, the pain goes away completely and leaves in its wake a feeling of euphoria. This phase after the attack is called postdrome.

DO MIGRAINES OFFER AN EVOLUTIONARY ADVANTAGE?

Migraine is very disabling, but it's part of the genetic code of more than 10 percent

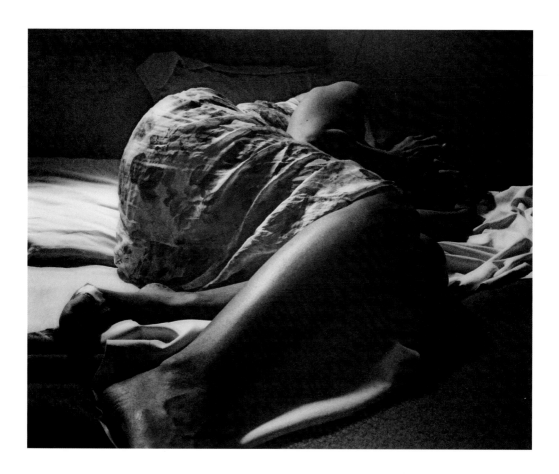

of human beings. Could there be an evolutionary advantage to having migraines? At least two theories may be put forward on this subject. First, since migraine sufferers have hypersensitive brains, they may have the advantage of perceiving information imperceptible to other individuals. In the past, that may have been an advantage in avoiding certain threats. What's more, since a migraine attack can indicate a metabolic imbalance, it forces the sufferer to take refuge in a protected resting place. This behaviour may have had positive consequences for the preservation of some individuals. Obviously, today, the very high level of stimulation in our environment can be intolerable for migraineurs and attacks have predominantly negative effects on how they function.

In summary, it can be said that migraine is the manifestation of a cerebral state of altered excitability able to activate the trigeminal-vascular system in response to metabolic imbalances or external stimuli. This biological sensitivity is determined by a number of genes. The intracranial neurogenic inflammation triggered then causes migraine pain that can be felt in the head or the neck. The brain disruptions related to the attack explain the many accompanying symptoms. The best way to study migraine is still to gather descriptions of migraine sufferers' symptoms and try to understand them in a scientific way.

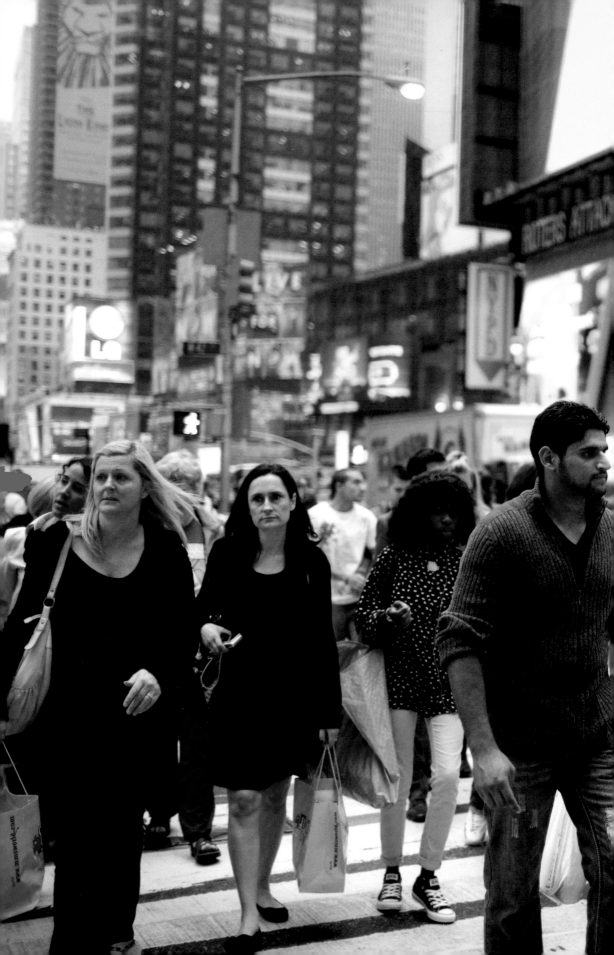

CHAPTER 4

Categories of Migraine and Links to Other Diseases

There are, in truth, no specialties in medicine, since to know fully many of the most important diseases a man must be familiar with their manifestations in many organs.
— Sir William Osler

Migraine is a disease with a thousand faces (see page 74). It can almost be said that there are as many different kinds of migraine as there are migraineurs, since every brain is unique. Symptoms vary, attack frequency varies, triggers vary, and so do coexisting diseases. All of these variations sometimes make diagnosing and treating migraines complicated. This chapter outlines the categories of migraines and the various medical conditions that may accompany and influence them.

MIGRAINE TYPE BY ATTACK FREQUENCY

Migraine frequency is a continuum. During their lifetime, migraineurs may experience episodic and chronic periods, depending on their state of health and how well they are functioning. In some cases, migraines may disappear for years, which can be considered a remission. People who have episodic migraine attacks have a 2.5 percent chance per year of developing a chronic form of the disease. Conversely, those with chronic migraine will return to an episodic state a year or two later in 26 percent of cases. In a small number of patients, chronic migraine may persist for years and severely affect quality of life. When this situation continues despite attempts at treatment, it's called refractory migraine. But first let's define the terms "episodic" and "chronic."

EPISODIC MIGRAINE

The vast majority of migraineurs experience clearly defined attacks with migraine-free intervals (Figures 24 and 25). Most days go by normally, without headache. The onset of the attack is easily recognized, so keeping track of the number of attacks per month in a diary is simple. Those who have fewer than fifteen headache days per month have episodic migraine. The figure of fifteen days per month is completely arbitrary, however — remember that we're talking about a continuum, not sharply divided categories. Even in the episodic category, cases

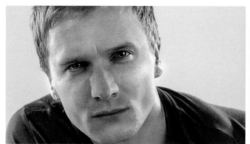

Paul, 24
**Asthma
Epileptic mother
Migraine with aura
Four attacks a year**

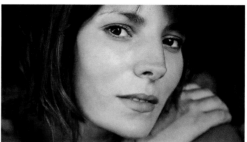

Cynthia, 32
**Difficult childhood
Fibromyalgia
Depression
Episodic migraine**

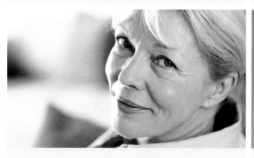

Claire, 62
**High blood pressure
Menstrual migraine from age fifteen to fifty
Stopped at menopause**

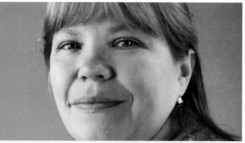

Nancy, 40
**Obese
Sleep apnea
Car accident
Chronic migraine**

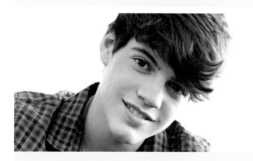

Gabriel, 14
**Motion sickness at age six
Mother with migraines
Soccer concussion
Monday migraine**

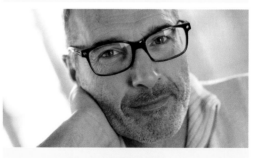

Damian, 50
**Anxiety disorder
Obsessive traits
Sleep disorders
Frequent episodic migraine**

↗ A Thousand Faces: Patient Files

are very diverse: some people have a few attacks per year in exceptional circumstances. Others have more frequent attacks: one or two per week, for example. Sometimes this group (seven to fourteen headache days per month) is labelled "frequent episodic." Some experts think that frequent episodic migraineurs should be treated in the same way as chronic migraineurs, since the impact of their migraines on their quality of life is similar. The severity of the attacks may also vary. A headache treated in under an hour is a lot different from a severe attack lasting three days!

CHRONIC MIGRAINE

Chronic migraine is a severe form of the disease, affecting between 1 and 2 percent of the population in most countries. Someone with chronic migraine has headaches more than half the time, and sometimes even every day. Chronic migraine has been described fairly recently in the

MIGRAINEURS: THERE ARE SEVERAL SUB-GROUPS

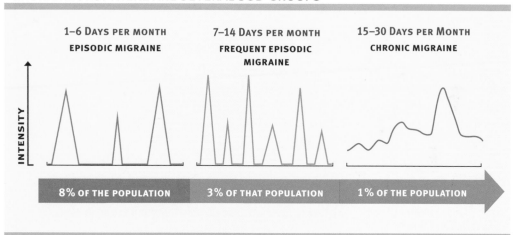

FIGURE 24

EPISODIC AND CHRONIC MIGRAINE

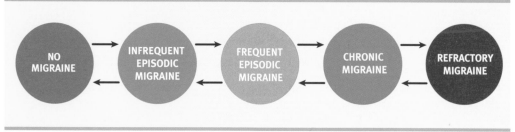

FIGURE 25

75

scientific community and the diagnosis is often unfamiliar to doctors, quite simply because most of them have not learned how to recognize or identify it during their medical training. An exact definition of chronic migraine is very important since a clear definition allows scientists to study this particular category of patients and develop suitable treatments.

In general, people with chronic migraine have varying degrees of headache that can often be divided into three categories, depending on their impact on activities and the severity of the symptoms (Figure 26). Mild headache, or "background headache," is very frequent, perhaps even constant, but it does not always develop into an attack. It may be accompanied by pain or stiffness in the neck. Other migraine symptoms, like nausea and photophobia, are absent or very mild. Usually, at this level, the person can function, as the pain is "annoying, but not strong." During a moderate attack, the headache's intensity increases, and migraine symptoms are more noticeable. It's nonetheless still possible fo those affected to maintain your activities, even if less effectively. Finally, when the attack becomes severe, the pain and related symptoms are so intense that activities have to be stopped, and the person has to lie down or at least be alone. Severe attacks may last several days and often do not respond to any treatment.

MIGRAINE HEADACHES: LEVELS OF SEVERITY

Mild or Background	Moderate	Severe
The pain is frequent, even daily, and mild.	The intensity increases.	The pain is severe.
Migraine symptoms are absent or not very intense.	Migraine symptoms are present.	Migraine symptoms are severe.
Activities are possible.	Activities are slowed down.	The patient must lie down or be alone.
Treatment is not always necessary.	Treatment is necessary.	Treatment is necessary and may fail.

FIGURE 26

CHRONIFICATION FACTORS

Certain factors have been associated with the transformation of episodic migraine into chronic migraine: being female, obesity, sleep apnea, past head or neck trauma, regular caffeine consumption, and more frequent migraines in the preceding year (Figure 27). The onset of severe attacks early in life has been reported as a poor prognostic factor. Physical or sexual assaults during childhood are associated with chronification, but are also related to other factors such as anxiety and depression. The existence of other painful disorders also increases the likelihood of more frequent migraine attacks. According to some researchers, the most frequent combination leading to migraine chronification begins with a stressor that first causes sleep disorders, then anxiety, and then medication abuse (Figure 28). Increasing attacks, deteriorating sleep and chronic stress may trigger muscle tension in the neck and jaws that can also help perpetuate the cycle.

Joanne, 45

Joanne's neurologist asked her how many migraines she had every month. She thought for a moment, and then replied: "Six or seven, at least I think so...." The doctor then asked her how many days a month she didn't have any headache at all. Joanne realized that it was hard for her to imagine a day without a headache. Of course, she had more severe attacks, but she also had less intense headaches in between. For her, these headaches were almost "normal." When she counted all the headaches, the total came to twenty-five days per month.

Even though the association between these factors and chronic migraine is known, it hasn't yet been solidly demonstrated that treating reversible factors (like sleep apnea or caffeine overconsumption) leads

MIGRAINE CHRONIFICATION RISK FACTORS

Age	Frequent Attacks Initially
Low Socio-Economic Level	Obesity
Head Trauma	Overconsumption of Medications
Other Painful Disorders	Stressful Events
Poorly Managed Medical Conditions	Regular Caffeine Use
Predisposing Genes	Sleep Apnea

FIGURE 27

Adapted from M.E. Bigal and R.B. Lipton, *Headache*, 2006.

to an improvement where migraines are concerned. Most headache clinics work on these aspects to try and interrupt the vicious cycle.

MEDICATION-OVERUSE HEADACHE

We can't talk about chronic migraine without tackling the subject of medication overuse (Figure 29). These infamous "rebound headaches" are associated with frequent migraines. Almost half of chronic migraineurs may experience medication "abuse," by medical standards. What constitutes abuse varies with the substance in question. For acetaminophen and anti-inflammatories, the limit is set at fiteen days a month. For triptans and narcotics (like morphine and codeine), it's set at ten days a month. For a combination of treatments, the limit is also ten days per month. This means that if you

have fewer than eight headache days per month, you're at low risk of developing a medication-overuse headache, even if you treat all your headaches.

What causes rebound?

The brain is a constantly changing and constantly adapting organ. However, it doesn't always adapt the way we might want. We might dream about an ideal situation in which the brain, exposed to frequent migraine attacks, would generate natural mechanisms to block them and make the sensory system less sensitive, more resistant. Unfortunately, the exact opposite happens. The closer together the migraine attacks are, the more sensitive the system becomes, meaning that attacks are triggered more and more easily. A lowering of the migraine threshold is sometimes talked about, as if the bar for the onset of an attack

A VICIOUS CYCLE

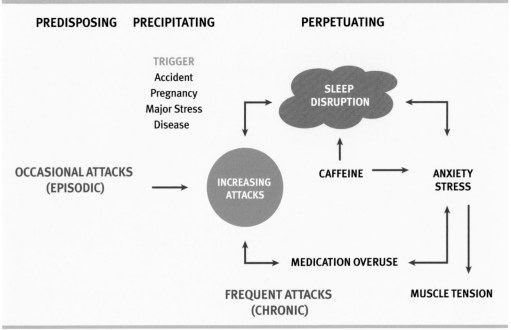

FIGURE 28   Adapted from Dr. Anne Calhoun.

Josie, 52

In her twenties, Josie had a few migraines every year. After her second pregnancy, she had a depressive episode. During this period, her migraines were much more frequent: she slept very badly and experienced a great deal of anxiety trying to juggle family and work. In her forties, things got better, but following a car accident, the attacks increased. She began to have almost constant neck tension and now has migraines more than ten days a month.

Josie has tried to see a doctor, but the waiting lists are long. In the past six months, she has often taken acetaminophen, saving her triptans for "real attacks." Since acetaminophen has little effect, she often winds up taking a triptan, which has become less effective because she's taken it too late. She has trouble getting over her long attacks, and on the rare days without attacks, she catches up late on work. Of course, she now drinks four cups of coffee a day to "make it through the day," and she's having trouble sleeping again. After meeting with a neurologist, she's planning withdrawal, but she's worried: how will she be able to do without her medications?

MEDICATION OVERUSE:
A CHRONIFICATION RISK FACTOR

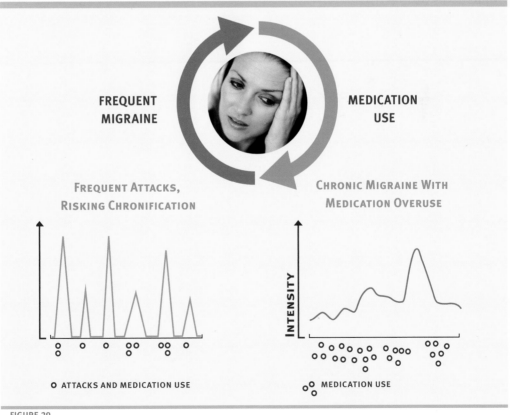

FIGURE 29

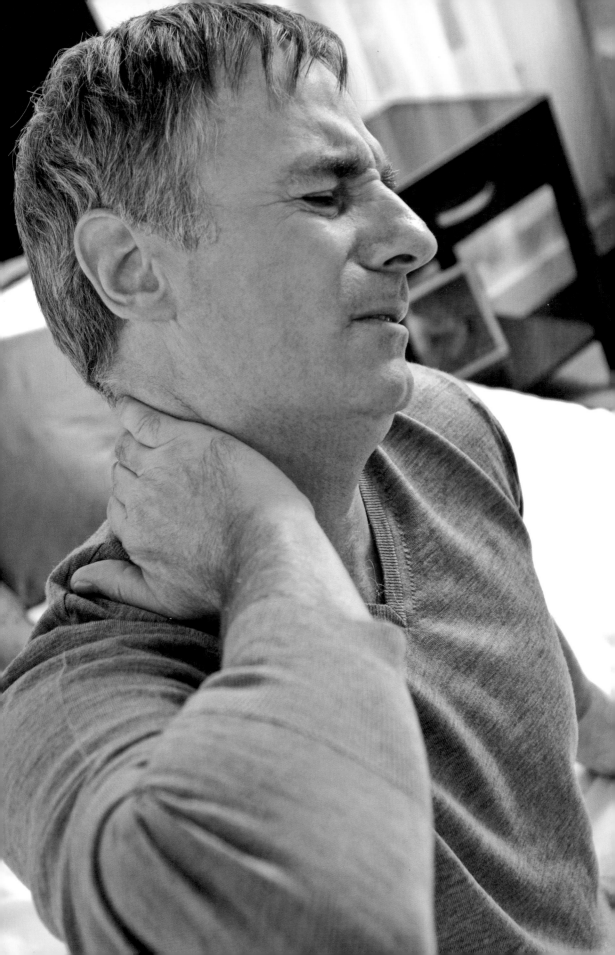

The Fiorinal Story

The first clinic to specialize in headaches was established in the 1940s at the Montefiore Medical Centre, by Dr. Arnold Friedman. While this famous clinic was able to help and continues to help a great many people, its history is nonetheless linked to medication-overuse headache. In fact, Fiorinal, a product containing aspirin, caffeine, and butalbital, sometimes combined with codeine, was developed by Dr. Friedman and named after his clinic. Triptans did not exist at the time, and migraineurs very often just had to put up with their attacks. This product very quickly became a great success with migraine sufferers for treating attacks. Butalbital, a barbiturate, is a treatment for anxiety and no doubt contributed to the well-being felt by anxious migraineurs. But it was soon observed that regularly consuming caffeine and barbiturates led to chronification. The result was that Fiorinal became enemy No. 1 for headache specialists, sometimes to the great despair of patients who had fallen into the trap of medication-overuse headache. Since 2013, the American Headache Society has recommended not using barbiturates or narcotics to treat migraines.

were set lower and lower. On the microscopic level, this sensitization is found at every level of the brain's electrical network: the cortex is more sensitive, the thalamus is more sensitive, the brain stem is more sensitive, and so are the sensory nerves. Regularly taking medications contributes to this phenomenon. The brain gets used to painkillers and responds less and less, meaning that stronger, more frequent doses are needed. At the extreme, some people have to take very high doses of several medications every day to prevent headache. Very often, these people have a constant mild headache, sometimes worse in the morning, and medications just prevent the onset of a more severe attack, without really relieving the pain.

What do we mean by a withdrawal process?
Withdrawing from medications is like resetting the organism. Stopping the consumption of medications is an attempt to return the neurons to the way they functioned initially. Obviously, withdrawal can cause headaches, sometimes severe and lasting several days. This is usually a painful stage for a migraine sufferer. Again, minimum withdrawal time varies depending on the substances taken, but usually it's estimated to take from three to four weeks for withdrawal to be deemed a success. Many people get discouraged after a week, which is not long enough for them to improve. Withdrawal can be made easier by taking certain medications to manage the rebound, but patients must discuss this with their doctor. That said, no totally effective treatment has yet been discovered to manage withdrawal. It's also important to know, without getting discouraged, that withdrawal is not universally effective either. Nearly half the time, migraines remain frequent after

withdrawal, and other treatments must be tried to manage them. In this situation, it's assumed that medication overuse was not the main cause of the chronic headaches. There is therefore a distinction between medication overuse as such and medication headache caused by overuse. If this distinction between concepts puzzles you, you should know that most doctors also find this a difficult subject. Taking medications regularly, triptans included, may in some cases remain the only way to have an acceptable quality of life, but this conclusion should never be reached before a proper withdrawal process has been completed. Of course, relapse is always possible, especially if the migraines are hard to manage and remain frequent.

THE REPERCUSSIONS OF CHRONIC MIGRAINE ON MOOD AND QUALITY OF LIFE

Chronic migraine sufferers are at higher risk for anxiety or depression disorders (Figure 30). There is also an association with bipolarity and certain personality disorders. People with chronic migraine use more sick leave than those with episodic migraines. Their migraines are very disabling, and they often have to deal with the fact that their difficulties are not recognized. Family and friends have trouble believing that their attacks are so frequent and sometimes get tired of hearing repeated complaints. "Change the CD! We never go out anymore! When are you going to feel better?"

PREVALENCE OF ANXIETY AND DEPRESSION BY MIGRAINE SEVERITY

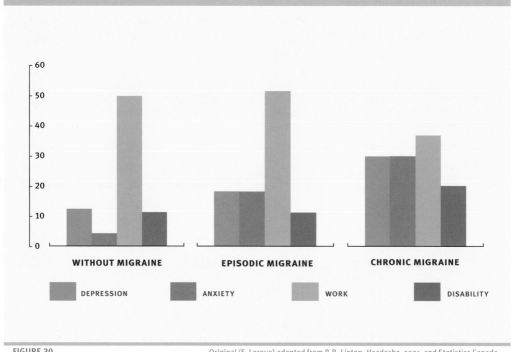

FIGURE 30   Original (E. Leroux) adapted from R.B. Lipton, *Headache*, 2001, and Statistics Canada.

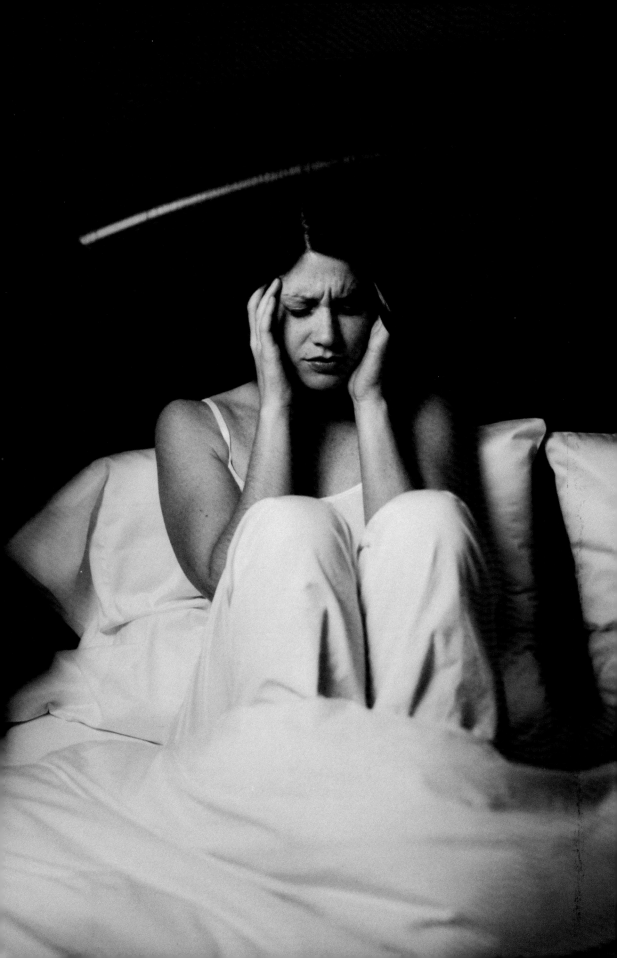

REFRACTORY MIGRAINE

According to the *Oxford English Dictionary*, the term refractory means "obstinate, stubborn, unmanageable, rebellious." Most chronic diseases, like asthma and epilepsy, have refractory forms that are hard to treat. A precise definition of refractory migraine is a work in progress. It's a subcategory of chronic migraine, characterized by frequent severe attacks with a major impact on quality of life, and not improving even after several treatments have been tried. This form of migraine is almost always accompanied by mood and sleep disorders. Even among this severely affected subgroup, there is a continuum of severity based on the impact on functioning: a refractory migraine sufferer may be able to work full-time or part-time, or may be disabled.

The cause of refractory migraine has not yet been precisely determined. The same mechanisms that lead to migraine chronification are no doubt involved, but in a continual and severe form. For example, a migraine attack is triggered by an imbalance in neuronal activity, but eventually equilibrium is re-established. It's possible that the brain of a refractory migraine sufferer is in a perpetual state of imbalance and that the pain control pathways are never adequate. It's also possible that a

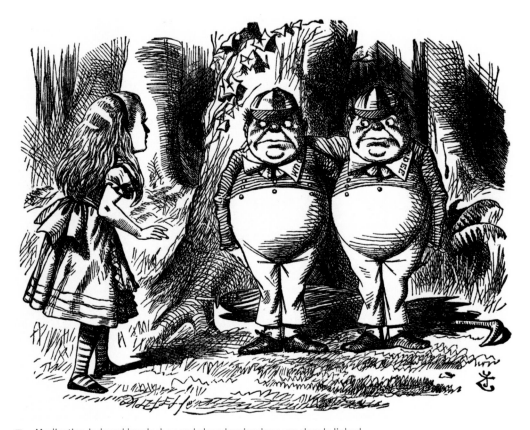

↗ Medication-induced headaches and chronic migraines are closely linked.

"persistent trigger" causes brain imbalance and generates continuous attacks. People with refractory chronic migraine often report persistent allodynia (or hypersensitivity of the skin) and a constant hypersensitivity to sounds, smells, or light. They often describe unending neck pains that may trigger attacks, but don't disappear once the attack is over.

Managing refractory migraine is a considerable challenge for both doctor and patient. It requires a lot of time, scientific rigour, empathy, and listening. Patients with refractory migraine justifiably get discouraged; they are sometimes exhausted and worried, and may react to their difficult situation in many ways — with anger, by casting doubt on treatment, and with passivity. A multidisciplinary approach is recommended but seldom available. Treatment for refractory migraine is based on the same principles as for migraine in general: good lifestyle habits, optimal use of acute treatments, monitoring of medication overuse, treatment of related diseases, and management of mood and sleep disorders. In addition, people with refractory migraine often feel a lack of recognition and understanding from those around them. In contrast to people with cancer, for example, who are looked after by teams and encouraged by family and friends to "fight to be cured," migraine patients are often told to "accept" their condition and receive relatively little support. This situation is bound to change as a result of scientific advances in understanding migraine mechanisms. The better the disease is understood, the more effective treatments will be, and the less migraine will be considered a benign and unimportant disease.

MIGRAINE WITH AURA

Aura is a visual phenomenon described in detail in Chapter 3. The international classification contains a specific category for migraine with aura, but this classification does not take into account the wide variation in the frequency of auras in migraine sufferers. Indeed, some people only have migraines with aura, as if this were their only trigger. These people may experience a flurry of auras — a large number of auras in a short period of time. Others have migraines without aura, but experience a few auras each year. Finally, it's even possible to have auras without a headache; this is often observed in people fifty and over. Given this knowledge, the often-used term "ophthalmic migraine" should be abandoned.

MENSTRUAL MIGRAINE

The menstrual cycle influences migraines in most women. Almost 60 percent of female patients report that the attacks that occur during their menstrual periods are the most intense, last longer, and are harder to treat than others (Figure 31). These attacks may recur several days in a row. Menstruation is associated with a decrease in blood estrogen levels, and it's clear that this drop influences the brain and promotes the onset of attacks. What's more, menstruation has an inflammatory aspect, as the uterus sheds its lining, causing bleeding. The rise in prostaglandins related to this inflammation can cause the abdominal cramps familiar to many women, but also trigger a migraine attack.

We talk about pure menstrual migraine when attacks occur only during the menstrual period, and about menstrual-related migraine when attacks not related to the menstrual period also occur. Women for whom there is a clear connection between their periods and their migraines will have a better chance of seeing their condition improve during pregnancy, when estrogen levels stabilize, and at menopause, when hormonal cycles stop. This sensitivity of the brain to hormones may also be caused by genetic factors. Treating menstrual migraine is sometimes quite a challenge. A number of specific approaches can be used, for example, taking an acute migraine treatment regularly for a short time around the menstrual period, known as mini-prophylaxis. Uninterrupted use of oral contraceptives is sometimes recommended, but must be discussed with a doctor.

CHILDHOOD MIGRAINE EQUIVALENTS

Children may have migraines, but a number of other childhood disorders are also linked to the onset of migraines in adulthood. These syndromes usually occur as attacks, just like migraines, and are called "childhood migraine equivalents." In some cases, they are also seen in adults. Symptoms include cyclic vomiting, abdominal migraine, paroxysmal vertigo, and spasmodic torticollis. Colic and motion sickness have also been associated with migraines. Cyclic vomiting syndrome can also occur in adults. The vomiting episodes recur several times a year, last a few days, and may require hospitalization. Often, many gastroenterological tests are carried out before a diagnosis is made. Some anti-migraine treatments may be useful in treating this syndrome.

MENSTRUAL MIGRAINE

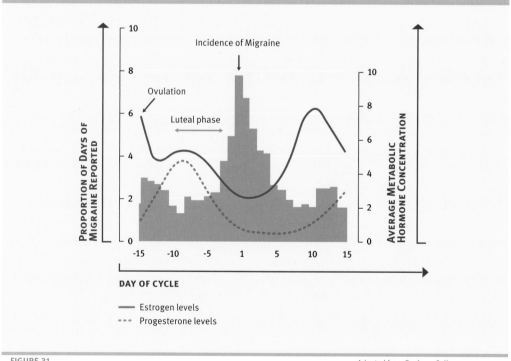

FIGURE 31

Adapted from Dr. Anne Calhoun.

The Many Roles of an Attack Diary

The main tracking tool for migraine attacks is a diary. Keeping a diary achieves several objectives and makes decision-making much easier for both patient and doctor. It gives us a handle on the situation. While at the beginning, most patients find keeping a diary restrictive, they later realize that it does have advantages. You don't have to keep an uninterrupted diary for years on end! Once you have answers to the questions asked, you can stop keeping it, and need only start again if your condition seems to get worse. Remember that in the world of migraines trends are seen over periods of two or three months and not two or three weeks.

The objectives of an attack diary:

1. Determine the frequency of attacks, by intensity.
2. Note the relationship between attacks and menstrual periods, if applicable.
3. Observe the effect of various triggers.
4. Determine which acute treatment works best.
5. Show the effectiveness of a preventive treatment.
6. Detect medication overuse and aid in appropriate withdrawal.

There are a number of ways to keep an attack diary. Most migraine clinics have their own format. Be sure you're comfortable with the tool used. Virtual diaries in smartphone apps, for example, are interesting, but sometimes hard for doctors to consult and file. Some people store their information on their telephone and then recopy the essential data into a paper diary (Figure 32).

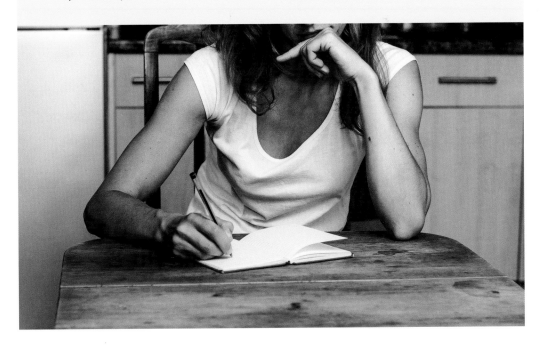

MIGRAINE AND OTHER DISEASES

The brain, whether that of a migraine sufferer or not, is affected by its environment (Figure 33). It's sensitive to what's happening inside and outside the body, and modulates its activity to suit the tasks to be done. To function, it depends on the ingredients it receives via the blood, and therefore on body function as a whole. In return, the brain adapts our organism's activity based on the information it receives: digestion, heart rate, blood pressure, sleep, immune activity, etc. The brain is the body's orchestra conductor, ideally leading the entire body in harmony and constantly listening to the organs. The interrelationship between the body and the brain is fundamental to life, but is sometimes overlooked in a dualistic system that often tries to separate the two.

As we discussed in Chapter 3, the mechanisms that trigger a migraine attack are complex. Brain function is the source of these attacks. It's therefore not surprising that several medical conditions can influence migraines or be related to them. Repeated migraine attacks can in return influence body function and a person's mood. The chicken or the egg, the cause or the result — we don't yet have the answers, but relationships can be observed and analysed. The coexistence of two diseases in one person over and above statistical probability is called comorbidity (Figure 34). There may be several reasons for two diseases to occur in a single person or in a subgroup of people (Figure 35).

The main diseases statistically associated with migraine are summarized in Figure 36. These associations may be more

AN ATTACK DIARY, 1 MONTH OUT OF 3

	1	2	3	4	5	6	7	8	9	10	11	12	13	14	15	16	17	18	19	20	21	22	23	24	25	26	27	28	29	30	31
HEADACHE 1 2 3 (Degree of Severity)				2				3	3	2	1	1						3				2	2				1			1	
AURA																															
TRIGGER																		X													
MENSTRUAL PERIOD										X	X	X	X																		
TREATMENT Zomig				X				X										X													X
TREATMENT Naproxen									X	X	X											X	X			X					
EFFECT OF TREATMENT				0				0	+	+								+				0	+			+				+	

FIGURE 32

THE BRAIN IS INFLUENCED
BY ITS ENVIRONMENT

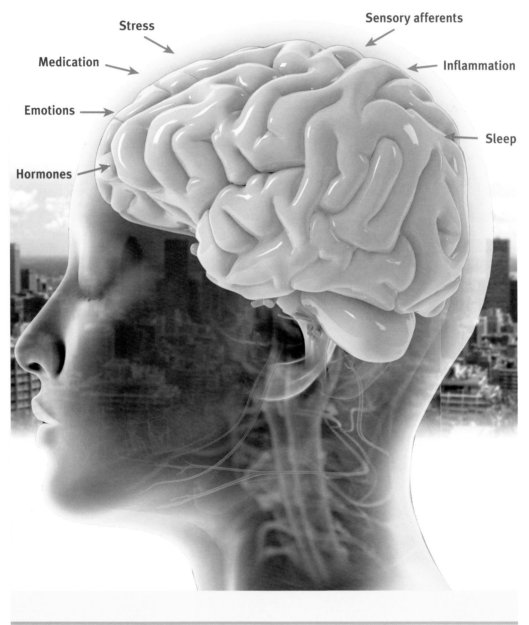

Stress

Sensory afferents

Medication

Inflammation

Emotions

Sleep

Hormones

FIGURE 33

WHAT IS COMORBIDITY?

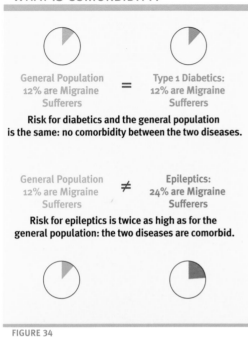

General Population
12% are Migraine
Sufferers

=

Type 1 Diabetics:
12% are Migraine
Sufferers

**Risk for diabetics and the general population
is the same: no comorbidity between the two diseases.**

General Population
12% are Migraine
Sufferers

≠

Epileptics:
24% are Migraine
Sufferers

**Risk for epileptics is twice as high as for the
general population: the two diseases are comorbid.**

FIGURE 34

or less obvious and more or less proven scientifically. For example, asthma is 1.2 times more common in migraine sufferers than in the general population, and the link is therefore minor. But epilepsy is twice as common among migraine sufferers and so the link is more significant. The link between two diseases can be observed either in a single direction or in both directions. Sometimes an association involves only a subgroup, and becomes stronger if the subgroup is the main focus of attention. For example, migraine is mildly associated with stroke (cerebrovascular accident or CVA), and this association actually only holds for migraine with aura, somewhat as if a very strong association in a small group became diluted in a larger

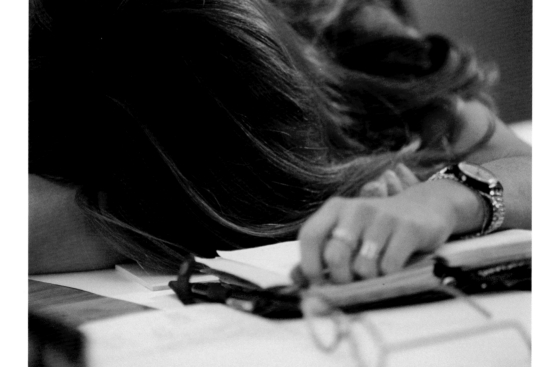

group. A great deal of caution must be exercised before making statements about the epidemiology of a disease, and especially about diseases defined solely on the basis of their symptoms, like migraine, depression, or dizziness. Figures on associations among diseases often vary depending on the study, and this is why they are not explained in detail here, to avoid inaccuracy or too long a list of results.

THE IMPACT OF COMORBIDITIES

Migraines cannot be treated in isolation from the rest of the body's functioning. First of all, a deterioration in the coexisting disease (asthma attacks, for example) can upset body metabolism and cause an increased number of migraines. As long as the asthma isn't under control, regaining control of the migraines will most likely be difficult. What's more,

COMORBIDITY : MIGRAINE AND DEPRESSION AS AN EXAMPLE

Cause of the Association	Description	Example
CHANCE	Diseases A and B are common and coexist in the same person with no biological connection.	Migraine affects 15 percent of women. Therefore, 15 percent of depressed women will also have migraines.
CONFUSION ABOUT THE DIAGNOSIS	A person has disease A, but because the symptoms look alike, receives a diagnosis of disease B.	Fatigue, insomnia, and loss of appetite are symptoms of depression, which can also be linked to migraines.
CAUSALITY	Disease A causes disease B.	Recurring migraine attacks cause depression.
COMMON MECHANISM	The same internal biological problem causes diseases A and B.	Migraine and depression are linked to serotonin metabolism.
GENETICS	Similar genes may influence diseases A and B.	Certain genes predispose people to both migraines and depression.
ENVIRONMENT	The same trigger causes diseases A and B.	A traumatic event may cause migraines and depression.

FIGURE 35   Adapted from R.B. Lipton, "Why are two diseases associated?" quoted by Mannix.

ANATOMY AND MEDICAL CONDITIONS

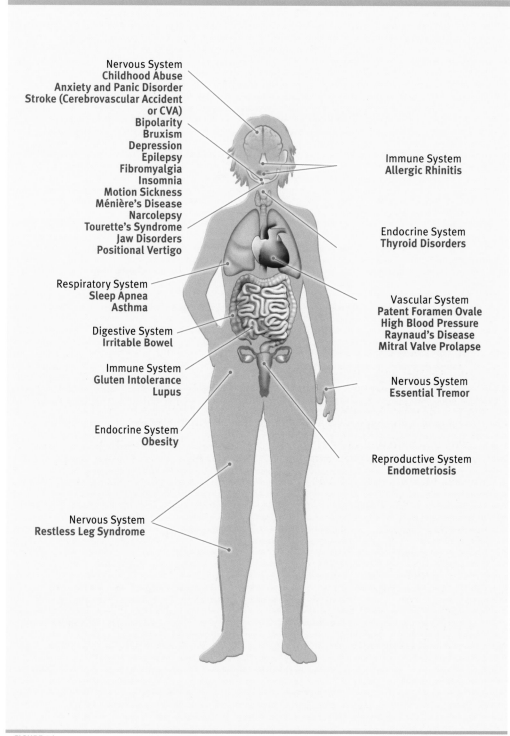

Nervous System
Childhood Abuse
Anxiety and Panic Disorder
Stroke (Cerebrovascular Accident
or CVA)
Bipolarity
Bruxism
Depression
Epilepsy
Fibromyalgia
Insomnia
Motion Sickness
Ménière's Disease
Narcolepsy
Tourette's Syndrome
Jaw Disorders
Positional Vertigo

Immune System
Allergic Rhinitis

Endocrine System
Thyroid Disorders

Respiratory System
Sleep Apnea
Asthma

Vascular System
Patent Foramen Ovale
High Blood Pressure
Raynaud's Disease
Mitral Valve Prolapse

Digestive System
Irritable Bowel

Immune System
Gluten Intolerance
Lupus

Nervous System
Essential Tremor

Endocrine System
Obesity

Reproductive System
Endometriosis

Nervous System
Restless Leg Syndrome

FIGURE 36

ELEMENTS DETERMINING QUALITY OF LIFE

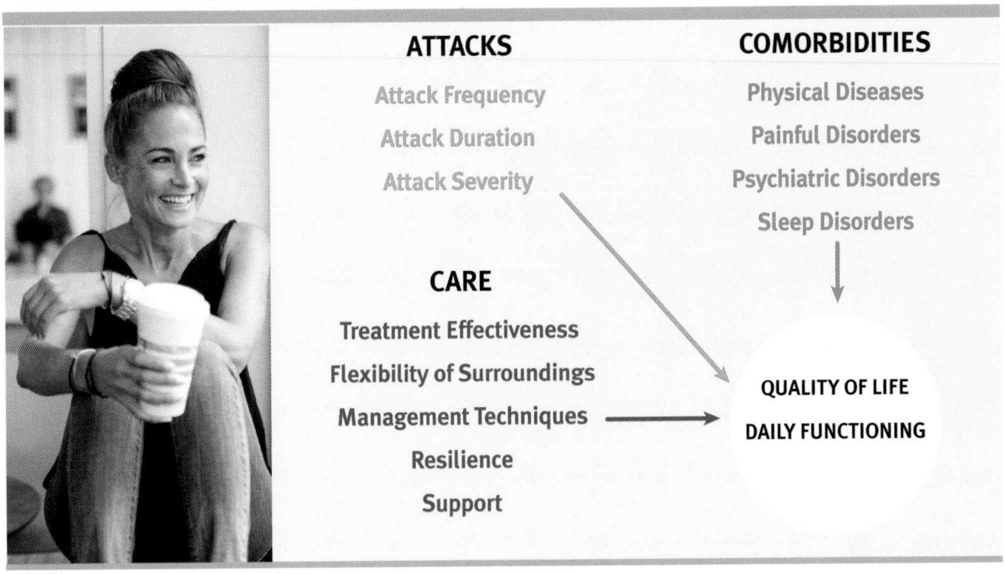

FIGURE 37

the various treatments used may have an impact on the comorbid disease. Someone with Crohn's disease, for example, cannot take anti-inflammatories, limiting the options for migraineurs who also have this disease. Conversely, it's sometimes possible to kill two birds with one stone and treat both diseases with the same medication, like the beta blockers used for high blood pressure that also treat migraines.

OVERALL FUNCTIONING

Diabetes treatment aims to avoid the long-term implications of hypergly-cemia. The main purpose of cancer treatment is to achieve remission and prolong life. Migraine is not a neurodegenerative disease, nor is it fatal. Thus, the ultimate goal of its treatment is to improve quality of life (Figure 37). When assessing a migraine sufferer, it's therefore essential to collect information on the frequency and severity of the attacks, but also on the state of the patient's physical and psychological health and overall functioning. Their environment, the people close to them and their workplace also have an impact on how to manage the attacks.

In the following chapters we will see that migraineurs have to play a role in their own care. They often have to demonstrate initiative, patience, resilience, and self-sufficiency. Only by taking all of these elements into account is it possible to improve the situation permanently.

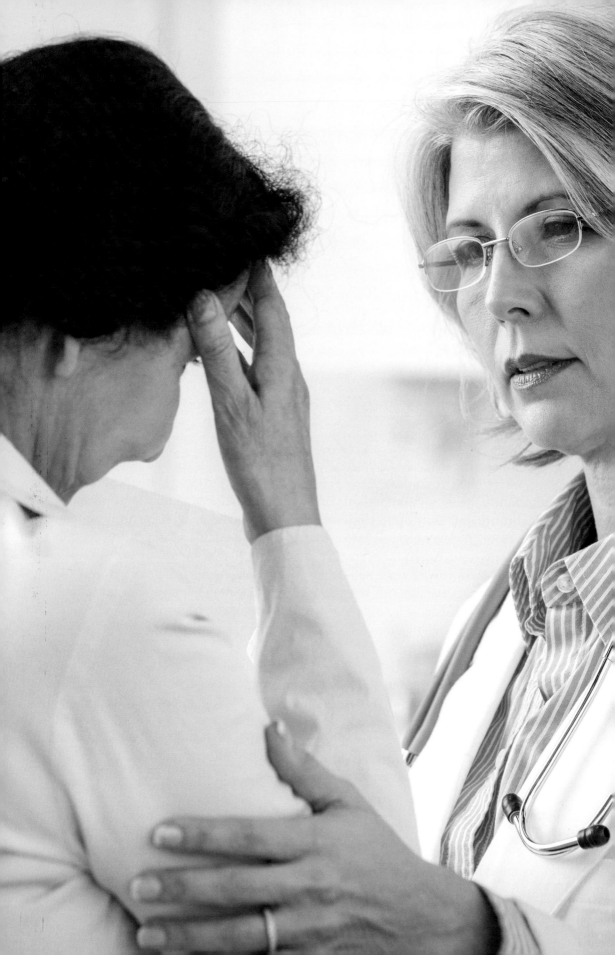

CHAPTER 5

Complex Therapeutic Choices

*No drug has yet been devised that permits the physician
to forget the importance of continued interest in the patient as a person.*

— Dr. John R. Graham

If you're a migraineur, you'd no doubt like to get rid of your migraines. Many patients are understandably very concerned about their future: Will I have migraines all my life? What can I do to have fewer of them? During their first medical consultation, many people jokingly say, "So, doc, am I going to have my head chopped off?" Obviously, there's no such thing as a "brain graft," nor is there a "100 percent effective medical treatment."

A predisposition to migraines is in part genetically determined and can't, therefore, at this point in time, be "cured." Nonetheless, the migraine brain's equilibrium can be improved using various approaches or even by natural biological evolution. The cessation of migraines at menopause in some women may seem like a "cure." When hormonal cycles are the main trigger for attacks, their cessation causes migraines to more or less disappear. But, in most cases, it's impossible to totally eliminate the attacks. Migraine is a brain dysfunction, and the brain is constantly interacting with its environment. Life is a moving equilibrium, and in migraine sufferers this movement may trigger attacks. Let's be honest: migraine has accompanied the human species for millennia; it's a painful, disabling, biological reaction, but one that's intimately linked to brain function. However, "learning to live with it" does not mean "enduring it without hope."

DOCTOR-PATIENT COMMUNICATION: A TALL ORDER!

Migraine management begins with a good therapeutic relationship between patient and therapist, whether this is a doctor or another professional. Several obstacles may arise between patients and doctors who try to communicate, and I think it's important to say a few words on this subject.

MEDICAL VOCABULARY

Doctors have a tendency to use medical jargon. They usually do so without realizing it. Medical training is based on learning a very precise scientific language. All medical students start their training with an ordinary vocabulary, used by the general public. Little by little, they have to learn to use medical terms. And believe me, they find this difficult! Years later, this specialized language will have replaced everyday language, and it's not always easy to switch from one to the other. If your doctor uses terms you don't understand, you must ask for them to be explained to you.

ANATOMICAL AND BIOLOGICAL CONCEPTS

Medical training requires memorizing the geography of the human body. The brain is especially complex, as it contains several small structures forming a compact mass and linked by many networks, a real muddle of connections. Migraine, too, is a complex phenomenon, located within this network. It's not always easy to explain these concepts as we would ideally like to, to be able to answer certain questions from patients on the nature of the disease.

LIMITED TIME

In an ideal world, doctors would have all the time they wanted to explain the mechanisms of the disease in detail to their patients and give them all necessary information on the prescribed treatments. But the fact is that available time is limited and, given the average length of fifteen minutes for family medicine appointments, explanations are often reduced to a minimum. Some diseases, like asthma and diabetes, have warranted the establishment of day centres or training centres for patients, so they can learn to better manage their disease. In Canada, this kind of facility doesn't yet exist for migraine. The doctor and patient thus have to make the most of the time available. It's often a good idea to prepare for a medical visit by bringing along a list of medications taken and your attack diary, and to write down your main observations or questions about recent medical symptoms.

EMOTIONS

When an episodic migraine sufferer discovers, on the suggestion of a doctor, an effective attack treatment, everyone usually goes home happy and satisfied. Patients see their quality of life improve and the doctor is pleased to have been able to help. But the problem is that some migraine sufferers don't find effective treatments in spite of all their efforts and those of their doctors. When pain won't go away, sleep is not restorative, medications produce side effects, and attacks occur repeatedly, it's normal to become irritable, even during a medical visit. As for doctors, they may feel powerless, discouraged and, not knowing what to do, they may also become impatient and irritable. In difficult moments like these, doctors have to remember one thing: the migraine sufferer's pain is real, and suffering patients, if they can't find an effective treatment, at least deserve a generous dose of support and sympathy. Patients have to remember that migraines are not the doctor's fault, and that anger and frustration can be harmful and exhausting. Managing emotions in cases of refractory migraine is a major challenge. Both sides must be aware of this in order to meet it.

HOW DO YOU CHOOSE THE RIGHT THERAPEUTIC APPROACH?

You've likely already looked for information on how to better manage your attacks (see image on page 98). During your search (and many patients describe a genuine obstacle course spanning years), you've no doubt experienced a number of classic challenges. First of all, you've had to juggle different pieces of well-intentioned, but not always effective, advice from those around you. According to your neighbour, your uncle, your work colleague, nothing could be easier than getting rid of your migraines! All you have to do is adopt this or that diet, consult such and such a chiropractor, and above all manage stress better. Second, you've perhaps had a lightning-fast meeting with a doctor who gave you medication, but without too many details on how to take it. On your follow-up visit, the treatment not having worked, you were perhaps told that there really is no other option and the best thing to do still is to learn to live with your attacks. The third situation involves enthusiastic recommendations from health professionals, promoting such and such a technique, manipulation, or this or that pillow or natural product, often at a considerable price. But the effects of these approaches are not always conclusive. Among the vaguely guilt-inducing recommendations of family and friends, the less than enthusiastic suggestions of doctors, and the promises of alternative medicines, how are you supposed to know which way to turn?

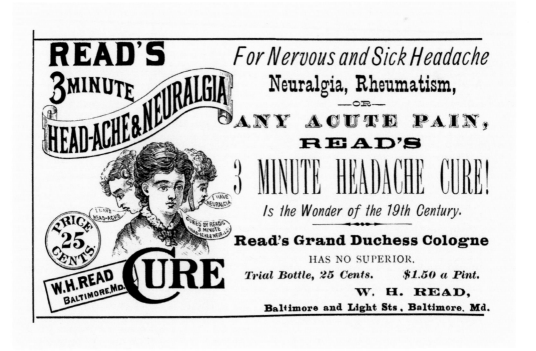

↗ There is no miracle treatment.

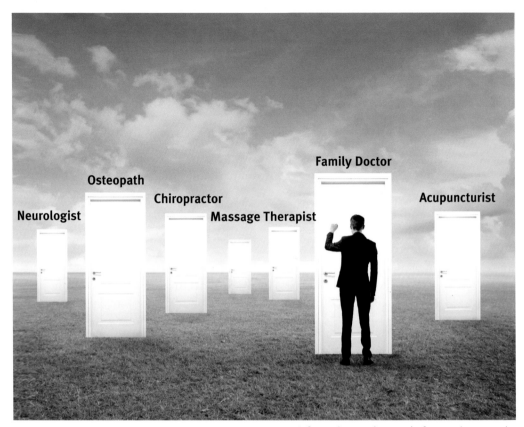

↖ Information can be sought from various people.

THE COMPREHENSIVE APPROACH TO MIGRAINE: THE THREE PILLARS OF TREATMENT

It's essential to keep in mind a few basic points about migraine, as illustrated throughout this book. First, migraine has existed for thousands of years, and, as we saw in Chapter 2, there is no lack of treatments, both simple and extreme.

We've described in detail how complex migraine is. Each migraine sufferer is different; each migraine sufferer is unique. Migraine management must take this diversity into account. The neurological processes causing migraine involve a great many receptors, proteins,

and neurotransmitters, in an equilibrium that varies with each person's genetic code and state of health. Medication A will be useful for and well tolerated by Melanie, but very poorly tolerated by Anne. There is thus no miracle drug and no "best" medication. Migraine triggers also vary from person to person. An approach focused on sleep will be miraculous for your friend, but you may need to work on neck posture instead.

The aim is to meet two objectives: to have the fewest attacks possible and to make them as short and non-disabling as possible. The comprehensive approach to migraine is based on the chronic disease management model, which includes managing lifestyle habits, controlling attacks, and reducing their frequency.

LIFESTYLE HABITS

Our brain is in constant contact with our environment through our five senses, but also through the foods we eat and the air we breathe. The way we manage our bodies and our emotions is fundamental to its functioning. Migraine is a brain dysfunction, probably triggered by neural network imbalances. Logically, lifestyle habits influence migraine attacks; they are thus the first stage in migraine management and undoubtedly the most important. Putting the migraine brain into an environment where it functions well leads in many cases to a decrease in the frequency of attacks. This approach may also

include withdrawal in the case of medication- overuse headache, and management of coexisting diseases, such as anxiety and sleep apnea.

ACUTE TREATMENTS

Acute treatments are those taken as needed to stop an attack as soon as possible. Taken too often, they can cause medication-overuse headaches. Several treatments exist, and can be used on their own or in combinations. If there are different kinds of attack, several strategies can be employed, until most of the attacks are under control.

PROPHYLACTIC OR PREVENTIVE TREATMENTS

Preventive treatments cause the frequency of attacks to decrease when they are very

THE THREE PILLARS OF TREATMENT

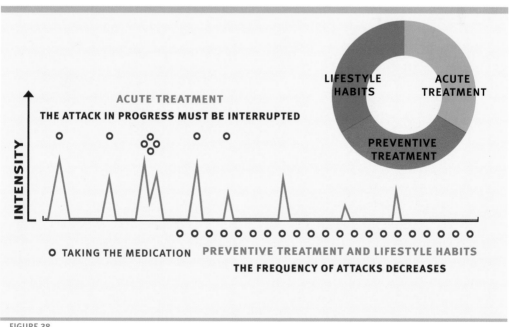

FIGURE 38

THE PLACEBO EFFECT

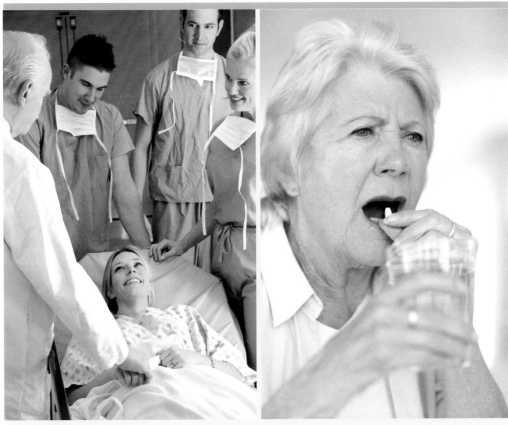

ATTENTIVE CARE
Sophisticated Treatment
High Expectations
Notable Placebo Effect

PATIENTS LEFT ON THEIR OWN
Simple Treatment
Few Expectations
Weak Placebo Effect

FIGURE 39

frequent. They modify brain function so as to raise the migraine threshold. They are therefore taken every day, regularly, whether the person is having an attack or not.

The distinction between an acute treatment and a preventive treatment is very important, but it isn't obvious to many patients starting out on their therapeutic journey (Figure 38). It's not uncommon in clinical practice to see someone taking an acute treatment every day or, conversely, a preventive treatment as needed. It's therefore very important for migraine sufferers to ask any questions they may have to make sure they fully understand the role of each drug.

A FEW BASIC CONCEPTS ABOUT MEDICATIONS

Every drug sold in Canada must first have been approved by Health Canada and have demonstrated its effectiveness and safety. Drugs always have two names, sometimes making the patient-doctor discussion more complicated. Each has a generic name, identifying the active pharmacological substance, and a brand name, used for marketing and sales. Very often, a doctor will ask how it's going with propranolol or Elavil, whereas the patient says she's taking Inderal or Apo-Amitriptyline. With the increasingly common use of generics, brand names sometimes get forgotten. When a product is generic, the name on the packaging is often preceded by the prefixes pro- or apo-, among others. In this book, the two names are presented in summary tables for greater clarity.

Drugs have important chemical characteristics that your doctor has to be familiar with and take into account when prescribing them. It's useful to know its absorption route (by mouth, by suppository, in an inhaler), speed of absorption, half-life (how long the medication remains in the bloodstream before it's eliminated from the body), interactions with other medications, and side effects. Each drug has a specific strength. A milligram of Dilaudid is not equivalent to a milligram of morphine! This is an important point, as some patients are fearful of the idea of taking three hundred milligrams of medication X, whereas for this particular drug this is a very low dose.

TREATMENT EFFECTIVENESS: SCIENTIFIC STUDIES, THE PLACEBO AND NOCEBO EFFECTS

RANDOMIZED CONTROLLED STUDIES

Given the abundance of alternative anti-migraine treatments offered by many sellers on the market, it's important to say a few words about the way doctors decide which treatments to suggest. When a product or a procedure is approved by Health Canada, it means that its effectiveness and safety have been demonstrated in what are called randomized control group trials. A random study is based on the principle of the control group, representing the disease's natural progression. Some diseases have a tendency to resolve themselves on their own after a period of time — this is in fact the case with a migraine attack. To determine a treatment's effectiveness, it must be compared with a placebo, an inactive substance. For example, if one hundred people with pneumonia are treated with an antibiotic and the results are compared with those of a hundred people given a sugar pill, then if the antibiotic is effective we should see that the health of the antibiotic group improves faster than that of the placebo group. These are usually double-blind studies, meaning that neither the patient nor the doctor knows which treatment was administered in order to decrease the placebo effect (see below). The groups are divided randomly.

THE PLACEBO EFFECT, FRIEND OR FOE?

The placebo effect is by definition a beneficial effect that doesn't stem from the chemical properties of a drug or the mechanical effect of a manipulation. It explains why a sugar pill or an injection of inactive saline solution, known as placebo treatments, has a positive effect. The placebo effect is influenced by the expectations of the person who receives the treatment, the way the placebo is administered, genetic factors, and the patient's age. Children are especially sensitive to the placebo effect. In terms of the treatment, the more invasive and impressive it is, and the more it raises patients' expectations, the greater the placebo effect will be. For example, treatments involving an injection or a bright red pill will be more effective than a little white pill that looks like a thousand others. The behaviour of the care provider is also very important. When the prescribing professional really believes in the treatment, the nurse will be more attentive and provide explanations, and the placebo effect will be activated (Figure 39). Genetic factors related to the placebo effect are being studied. Some researchers think that patients called "placebo responders," people who very easily activate a placebo response, should be excluded from studies, since they make demonstrating the effectiveness of products tested more difficult.

In the field of pain research, the placebo effect really can prove to be therapeutic. Our brain contains extremely powerful pain-control networks that switch on in certain circumstances: just think about those marathoners who manage to run in spite of a sprained ankle, or about soldiers fleeing the battlefield despite serious wounds. When a placebo is given to relieve pain, the brain activates what are called descending pathways, or brain networks that modulate the intensity of painful sensations coming from sensory receptors. In the case of a painful stimulus, pressure on

a finger, for example, the brain will modulate the pain's intensity.

Studies on migraine treatment, whether for an attack or for prevention, have all shown a significant placebo effect. In a review of seventy-nine studies on preventive treatments, the rate of response (50 percent or more improvement) was 46 percent for active treatments. The average for placebo responses was 26 percent but varied greatly depending on the kind of intervention. Oral placebos had a 22 percent response rate, while sham surgery or acupuncture on non-therapeutic points had rates of 58 percent and 38 percent respectively. This means that sham surgery could produce a higher response than a real drug (taking into account methodological bias, of course).

So it's understandable why so many alternative treatments may appear to be effective in managing migraines. A migraine sufferer who is afraid medications are dangerous will seek out a natural option, which will no doubt be presented as "100 percent effective" by a convinced and convincing person. If the treatment involves needles or an operation, the placebo effect will be very powerful. The effect of a treatment will also vary depending on how the product is presented and how it is perceived by the person treated. Part of the placebo effect is also caused by spontaneous improvements. Every migraine must come to an end, and the frequency of migraine attacks can decrease without any treatment. Since we often have a tendency to go to the doctor when the situation is at its worst, the improvement that follows is not necessarily due to the treatment but to a simple process of natural regression to the mean. Lifestyle habits may also be changed when an individual is taking a trial treatment and can contribute to improvement.

Some doctors dream about controlling the placebo effect. Wouldn't it be extraordinary to be able to order the brain to close the pain valves at will, just by using the power of the mind? As soon as the migraine attack started, we could activate the descending pathways and get on with our day. This is not yet possible, but it's a fascinating area of research.

THE NOCEBO EFFECT: SIDE EFFECTS GENERATED BY THE BRAIN

Since a sugar pill can produce good results owing to the placebo effect, would it be possible for the same sugar pill to produce negative effects, a sort of reverse placebo effect? This is indeed the case. Unpleasant symptoms caused by a neutral substance have been named the nocebo effect — the word "placebo" comes from the Latin verb placere, "to please," and "nocebo" from "nocere," to harm. Just like the placebo effect, the nocebo effect is influenced by people's expectations. In scientific studies, it has been observed that the more that possible side effects are explained to participants, the more they are experienced, even among patients receiving the neutral substance. People who tend to read all of the drug usage instructions and consult the Internet looking for rare or dangerous reactions will therefore be at greater risk of triggering a nocebo effect. It must be remembered that anxiety can cause many somatic symptoms, including dizziness, nausea, difficulty concentrating, and numbness. People who are worried at the idea of taking a new treatment will undeniably experience increased anxiety, and this may

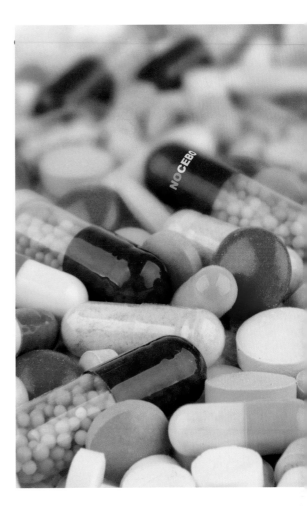

effect is, as a result, one of the causes of the many "intolerances" to medications. For this reason, it's sometimes better to persevere for a few days before you stop taking a medication; the undesirable effects may disappear.

DRUGS AND NATURAL PRODUCTS

Conventional drugs are sometimes badly perceived by the general public. The term "chemical" is often taken to mean "not natural" and therefore "dangerous." Some patients are afraid of disturbing their body's

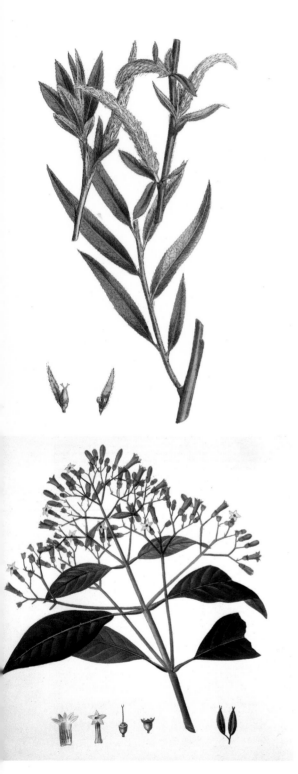

normal mechanism by ingesting pharmaceutical substances. Natural products are viewed as gentler, safer, and healthier. Furthermore, pharmaceutical companies are suspected (not always wrongly) of putting profit over health, which also makes people mistrust medications. If a drug is sold on prescription, it's often perceived as more dangerous. And the higher the cost of the medication, the more it's considered powerful and dangerous. This cost-related perception is especially true of triptans.

Yet for doctors and scientists in general, the difference between a natural product and a so-called "chemical" or "synthetic" substance seems very artificial. A product that effects the functioning of the human body is an active product, whatever its origin. In addition, several pharmaceutical products are in fact based on natural substances found in plants or produced by animals. Once the active chemical substance has been discovered, it's synthesized in a laboratory, making the commercial production of medications possible. Several examples of this can be given in the field of migraines. As for the safety of so-called "natural" products, it must be remembered that even the most powerful poisons and toxins we know about are entirely natural: the venoms secreted by snakes and spiders, as well as the poisons in some plants and mushrooms, are deadly. Lastly, some natural products are chemically similar to drugs and may interact with them, a known example being St. John's wort, used to treat depression, which interacts with antidepressants.

These perceptions about natural products play a very important and sometimes harmful role in migraine management.

↖ Above: *Salix alba* (salicin — anti-inflammatory).
Below: *Cinchona pubescens* (quinine — acetaminophen).

They may have the effect of scaring patients away from potentially effective treatments.

INTERVENTIONS THAT ARE DIFFICULT TO STUDY SCIENTIFICALLY

Doctors are far from being the only people trying to help those with migraine. A number of other healthcare professionals devote themselves to treating this common and painful disease. Among the specialties often called on for help are physiotherapy, osteopathy, chiropractic, acupuncture, massage therapy, psychotherapy, hypnosis, nutritional approaches, reflexology, and a large number of other alternative methods. These approaches are based on a wide variety of explanatory models for migraine. The role of the neck is central, according to therapies based on cervical manipulation, whereas intestinal inflammation and liver overload justify various diets.

This results in two phenomena doctors must be aware of. First, patients have several ways of explaining their migraine attacks, which significantly influences the choices made to manage them. They are hungry for information and are searching for the best treatments. The demand is therefore very high, given the number of migraine sufferers. Second, there are many alternative treatments, and they are often more accessible than an appointment with a doctor or at a migraine clinic. Some of these treatments are used with no solid scientific proof of their effectiveness. This situation may sometimes lead to unproductive discussions between a patient who is not completely satisfied with the approaches of traditional medicine and a doctor baffled by unfamiliar approaches.

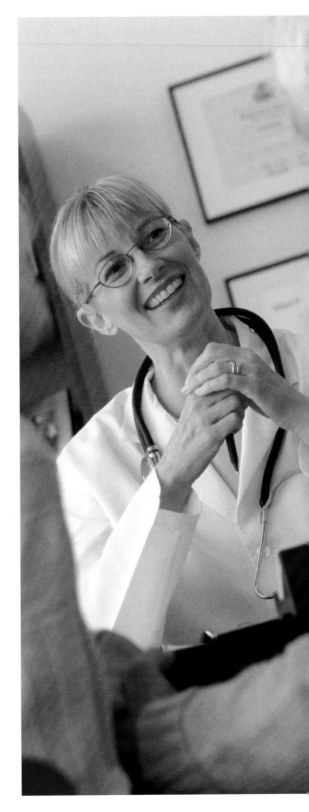

Some readers and therapists will perhaps be disappointed not to find in this book more details about the effectiveness of these approaches, but the author, being a doctor, doesn't have the required expertise to comment on these various treatments. What's more, there are so many techniques that an exhaustive and rigorous discussion of these approaches would take a whole book. It should however be remembered that for most of these techniques, no high-quality, randomized, double-blind controlled studies have been done, which means their effectiveness cannot be confirmed, at least according to medical standards. Treatments that have been the subject of scientific studies, in particular acupuncture and certain natural products, will be discussed in Chapters 7 and 8.

PREGNANCY AND BREASTFEEDING

Medications are never tested on pregnant women. This inevitably limits the options available during pregnancy and breastfeeding. The condition of more than 70 percent of women with migraines improves during their pregnancy, but the first trimester can be difficult. The use of non-pharmacological treatments (rest, cold compresses, relaxation techniques) is recommended as a first option. Acetaminophen and antinausea drugs are usually safe. Journal articles have been published to guide healthcare professionals in their recommendations. The use of any other drug should be discussed with a doctor.

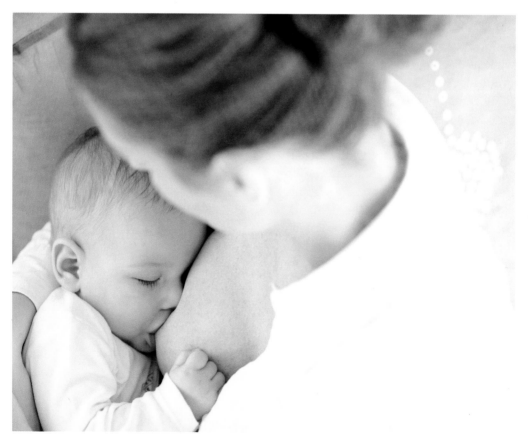

KEEPING AN OPEN MIND AND WORKING TOGETHER

Any discussion of treatments between a doctor and a patient must take into account what's known as the level of proof concerning any given therapy. What do we know about this treatment? How many people have tried it? What were the results? Were there any side effects? Was the product better than the placebo in the study? The problem with alternative treatments is that they haven't been studied in this way, with a few exceptions.

As doctors, we fear two things when a patient wants to try an alternative treatment. First of all, this treatment might be dangerous and harm the patient. Second, the treatment might be ineffective, and the costs incurred unjustified. Still, it's entirely possible that a treatment, even if it hasn't been recognized as effective, is associated with improvement in a condition, for three reasons. One, the disease may get better spontaneously. Two, the placebo effect may be triggered. Three, the treatment does indeed have a genuine physiological effect, but one that has neither been studied nor proven. In medicine, as in many other fields, the absence of proof is not the proof of absence!

Doctors must therefore keep an open mind. If patients want to try an alternative treatment, it's their choice, and the doctor's priority should be to ensure the safety of the treatment insofar as possible. Doctors should also remind themselves that the placebo effect can sometimes help the patient, and furthermore that some alternative treatments are perhaps effective, even though proof has not been established. In their communication with patients, they must use their knowledge to reassure and inform, not to force a choice or denigrate other approaches.

Patients must also keep an open mind. They have to try and understand why a doctor recommends one treatment and not another. They also have to be aware of the limits of knowledge about alternative treatments and beware of often expensive miracle solutions. And they have to confront their fears about traditional medicine.

In summary, on both sides, doctors and patients have to try to communicate their opinions and questions to each other. They should behave with respect toward each other, despite possible differences of opinion concerning alternative and traditional treatments. The common goal is to improve the patient's quality of life. The doctor always has a medical responsibility, but the final decision to take a treatment or modify lifestyle habits rests with the patient.

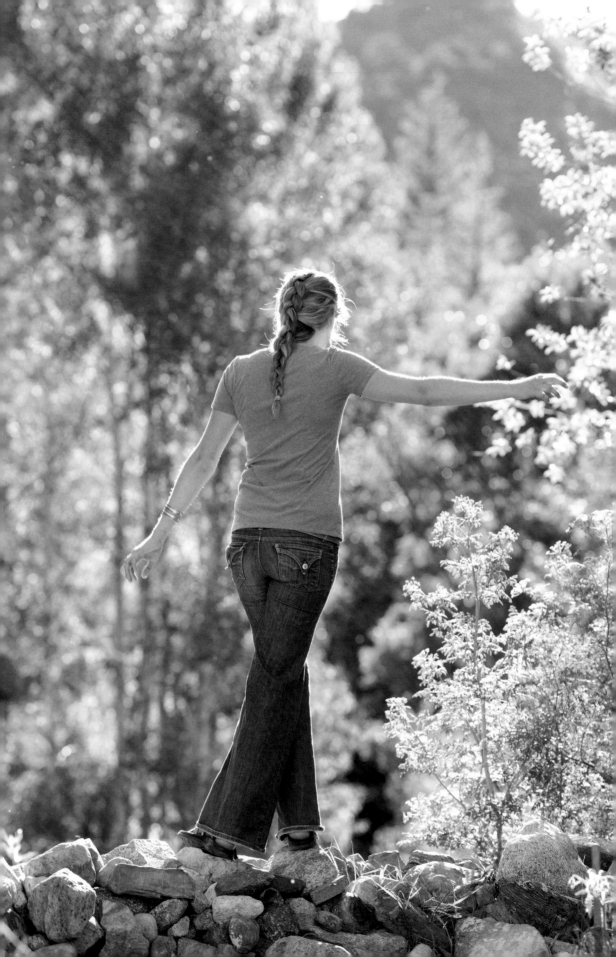

CHAPTER 6

Anti-Migraine Lifestyle Habits

For this the great error of our day in the treatment of the human body,
that physicians separate the soul from the body.

— Plato, *Charmides*

The migraine brain is sensitive to its surroundings. Sensations, biological information, emotions, perceptions, and chemical substances can all influence the brain and potentially cause an attack when a certain level of imbalance is reached. This makes it important for migraineurs to recognize their triggers and adopt a stable lifestyle. This step is often overlooked by doctors, although it's not very productive to try out an array of medications if lifestyle habits have not been modified.

ATTACK TRIGGERS

There are many possible triggers for a migraine attack (Figure 40). Some of them are cited by patients more often than others (Figure 41). Some triggers, like a drop in estrogen, alcohol, lack of sleep, and fasting, seem to be powerful enough to invariably result in an attack, but often a build-up of several triggers is required (Figure 42). Reliable scientific information on triggers is hard to come by, since they vary from one person to another and from one situation to another. Some triggers affect a large number of people in different ways; others are less widespread but almost always cause an attack in a particular person. Certain genetic factors likely play a role in sensitivity to one or another of these triggers, but no specific gene has yet been pinpointed. It must be stressed that some people, especially if they have very frequent attacks, tend to overestimate the number and role of triggers and fall into a cycle of avoidance that impairs their functioning even more than the migraines themselves.

ANTI-MIGRAINE LIFESTYLE HABITS

SLEEP
The links between sleep and migraines
We spend nearly a third of our lives sleeping. It's necessary for survival: extreme sleep deprivation causes hallucinations and may even lead to death. Nonetheless, despite the supposed improvement in quality of life in industrialized societies,

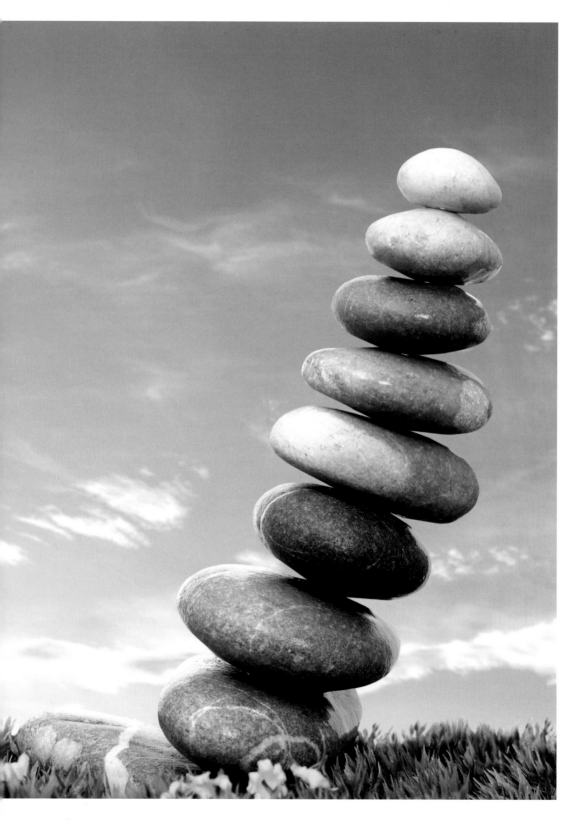

North Americans are sleeping on average two hours less each night in the 2000s than in the 1970s. Schedules are heavy, balancing family and work is difficult, and screen-based entertainment comes in many forms. The average Canadian spends no less than twenty-two to twenty-eight hours a week watching television, and digital screens are everywhere, preventing our brains from switching into "dark mode" in preparation for sleep.

There are many links between migraine and sleep. One of the great apparent paradoxes of migraines is that sleep can alleviate or trigger an attack.

Lack of sleep is a common and powerful attack trigger, cited by more than 40 percent of patients. Conversely, sleeping in later than usual may also contribute to the infamous weekend migraines — a dreadful kind of migraine that keeps sufferers from enjoying their days off. Irregular schedules, because of being on call or working night shifts, having young children or a partner who sleeps restlessly are all situations likely to cause increasingly frequent migraines.

Sleeping remains one of the classic treatments for relieving an attack. Patients often say that medications help, but until they've been able to sleep, the attack isn't really over. However, a significant percentage of migraines occur during deep sleep or in the early hours of the morning. Attacks occurring during the night or at dawn are often hard to treat, as the pain has already taken hold by the time the person wakes up. The tendency for migraines to begin during sleep becomes more pronounced with age; the percentage of migraine sufferers reporting these kinds of attacks rises from 16 percent for those in their twenties to 58 percent after the age of sixty.

Michael, 38

Michael's business is a great success. He doesn't keep track of the hours it takes to make it turn a profit. Long meetings, business trips, short nights, networking cocktails. In the past two years, Michael has noticed that his migraines have increased; he has them every week, and they slow down his activities. He's put on fifteen pounds and no longer works out. Since he eats a lot in the evening, he skips breakfast. Then he ends his day in front of his computer answering emails and has more and more trouble falling asleep. When his doctor pointed out to him that his lifestyle might contribute to his frequent migraines, Michael replied, "I know, but it's impossible for me to do things any other way!"

Several theories might explain this link between migraine and sleep. During deep sleep, we retain a certain amount of carbon dioxide, as breathing slows down. CO_2 is a powerful brain artery vasodilator, so it's possible that the vasodilation occurring naturally in some stages of sleep causes migraines. In addition, sleep is controlled by several areas in the brain stem located close to the nuclei responsible for migraine attacks. Greater electrical activity in these centres may trigger attacks.

Sleep disorders
Some sleep disorders, such as insomnia, restless legs syndrome, bruxism, and nightmares, are associated with migraines and other kinds of headache. Sleep apnea in particular has been linked to chronic migraine.

Chronic insomnia affects 10 percent of the general population, nearly 60 percent of those being monitored for a medical condition, and between 50 and 60 percent of migraine sufferers. Regular consumption of caffeine can make insomnia and anxiety worse, and cause a medication-overuse headache, with migraines triggered by mini-withdrawals.

Restless legs syndrome, or RLS, affects between 5 and 10 percent of the population and can seriously interfere with sleep.

Some studies suggest that this syndrome is associated with migraines. People with this problem describe unpleasant sensations in their legs when they are resting or close to falling asleep. These sensations may even be painful and make the person fidget and change position to seek relief. One of the causes of RLS is iron deficiency anemia, but several other causes are possible. Treatments do exist and a medical consultation is warranted if RLS symptoms have a negative impact on your quality of life.

MIGRAINE TRIGGERS

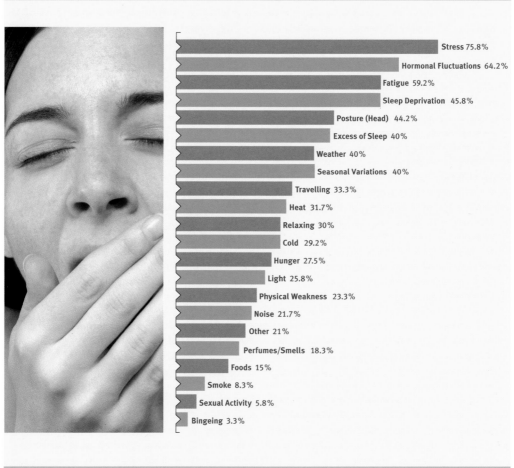

Stress 75.8%
Hormonal Fluctuations 64.2%
Fatigue 59.2%
Sleep Deprivation 45.8%
Posture (Head) 44.2%
Excess of Sleep 40%
Weather 40%
Seasonal Variations 40%
Travelling 33.3%
Heat 31.7%
Relaxing 30%
Cold 29.2%
Hunger 27.5%
Light 25.8%
Physical Weakness 23.3%
Noise 21.7%
Other 21%
Perfumes/Smells 18.3%
Foods 15%
Smoke 8.3%
Sexual Activity 5.8%
Bingeing 3.3%

FIGURE 40

Baldacci, *Headache*, 2013.

Nocturnal bruxism, or the tendency to tense the jaw or grind the teeth during the night, seems to be associated with migraines and may also cause tension-type headaches upon waking. A diagnosis of bruxism is not always easy to make, however, especially when the grinding is not audible. A dentist may notice excessive wear and tear on the teeth. In such cases, bite splints have been proposed as one way to reduce migraines, but they are not always effective.

Sleep apnea is a medical condition affecting from 10 to 15 percent of the population depending on the diagnostic, threshold chosen. Although we often think of someone with apnea as being an obese, snoring man, we mustn't forget that 25 percent of patients with apnea are women, between 10 and 20 percent are not obese, and between 10 and 20 percent don't snore! A short thick neck, a small chin and breathing through the mouth are other predictive factors for sleep apnea. While apnea

CATEGORIES OF TRIGGERS

HORMONAL FLUCTUATIONS	Menstrual period First trimester of pregnancy Perimenopause Contraceptives (very variable)
DIET	Skipping a meal, eating breakfast later Dehydration Caffeine withdrawal Alcohol, aspartame, monosodium glutamate, aged cheeses, chocolate, processed meats, citrus, etc.
STRESS AND STRONG EMOTIONS	Acute stress (accident, mourning, divorce, marriage, moving) Chronic stress (marital, professional, disease-related, financial) Drop in stress (weekend, holidays, professional deadline)
SENSORY STIMULI	Strong light Loud noises Odours (fragrances, gasoline, detergents)
SLEEP AND IRREGULAR ROUTINE	Lack of sleep Sleeping in, sleeping longer than usual Jetlag, travel Working variable shifts New baby
PHYSICAL ACTIVITY	Intense exercise Sexual activity
TEMPERATURE	Heat, humidity, changes in atmospheric pressure, chinook Smog, air quality

FIGURE 41

is not formally associated with episodic migraines, it's nonetheless a predictive factor for chronic migraines. It's also linked to morning headaches, which don't have the characteristics of migraines and tend to get better in an hour or two. If you feel sleepy during the day and have morning headaches, take it as a sign that you should undergo a screening test for sleep apnea. Sleep apnea also has significant effects on blood pressure and may play a role in heart disease. Finally, apnea doesn't just affect the person who has it, but also his or her sleeping partner: a study carried out by American researchers showed that spouses of snorers experienced poor quality sleep. As a result, it may be recommended to some patients to sleep in separate rooms a few nights a week to protect their sleep. This suggestion is not always welcomed with open arms, but it's an option to consider

if low-quality sleep and poorly controlled migraines are an issue.

Advice to promote sleep

Can the frequency of attacks be reduced by changing sleep habits? A very interesting study by Dr. Anne Calhoun attempted to answer this question. A group of patients with chronic migraine participated in a sleep study. The active group received five pieces of "real" advice (see Box on page 118), and the placebo group received "neutral" advice that in theory was not supposed to improve the subjects' quality of sleep. The result was encouraging! Overall, 35 percent of the patients who had received the real advice had fewer attacks, whereas not one patient in the control group had improved. Subsequently, both groups received real advice and, six weeks later, nearly half of the patients in each group had improved.

THE DASHBOARD: ADDING UP THE TRIGGERS

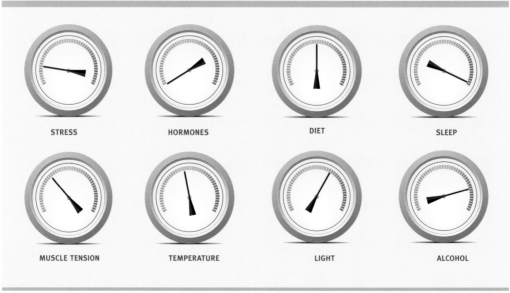

FIGURE 42

The researchers also observed that the more closely the patients followed the advice, the better their chances of improving their condition. They also noted that the consumption of painkillers had decreased significantly (patients had been given information about medication-overuse headache).

In conclusion, it's possible to reduce your migraines by improving sleep quality. Good sleep habits can be re-established in a few weeks, but in some cases professional support (cognitive-behavioural therapy) and temporary use of medications are necessary. There should be no chronic use of sleeping pills until sleep habits have been corrected. As with every therapeutic trial, a diary should be kept to observe the effect of the changes undertaken.

Diet

The impact of diet on migraines has a number of different aspects.

Obesity

A full-blown modern epidemic, obesity is responsible for 20 percent of deaths in western societies. Excess weight and obesity affect nearly two out of every three Americans. This fact also increasingly applies to children. Although obesity doesn't generally increase the risk of having migraines, people who are overweight or obese are at higher risk of having frequent or chronic headaches. One American epidemiological study showed that the risk of chronic headache was multiplied by three in obese people. Obesity affects our body in several ways. The posture of the spine changes; this can affect neck posture and cause pain, and therefore migraines. Fat maintains a state of chronic inflammation that might also cause attacks. Obesity is associated with

---

Five Things You Should Know About Migraine Attack Triggers

1. Everyone is sensitive to different triggers.
2. Triggers accumulate.
3. It's possible to have attacks with no obvious trigger.
4. A diary remains the best tool for detecting triggers.
5. Some triggers are beyond our control.

---

sleep apnea, itself linked to migraines. Last, obesity may increase intracranial pressure, possibly adding to the likelihood of frequent headaches.

Weight loss is a daily battle and concern for many North Americans. A few basic pieces of advice are suggested later in the chapter (Figure 43). The question of bariatric surgery naturally arises, given the increasing number of people undergoing it. A small series of studies suggests that this surgery may have a positive impact on migraines, but this operation is usually reserved for cases of morbid obesity and carries major risks. The effect of preventive medications on weight will be discussed in Chapter 8.

Fasting and dehydration

While several foods are often incorrectly singled out as migraine triggers, fasting and dehydration are often overlooked. It has been shown that these two metabolic states really do trigger attacks.

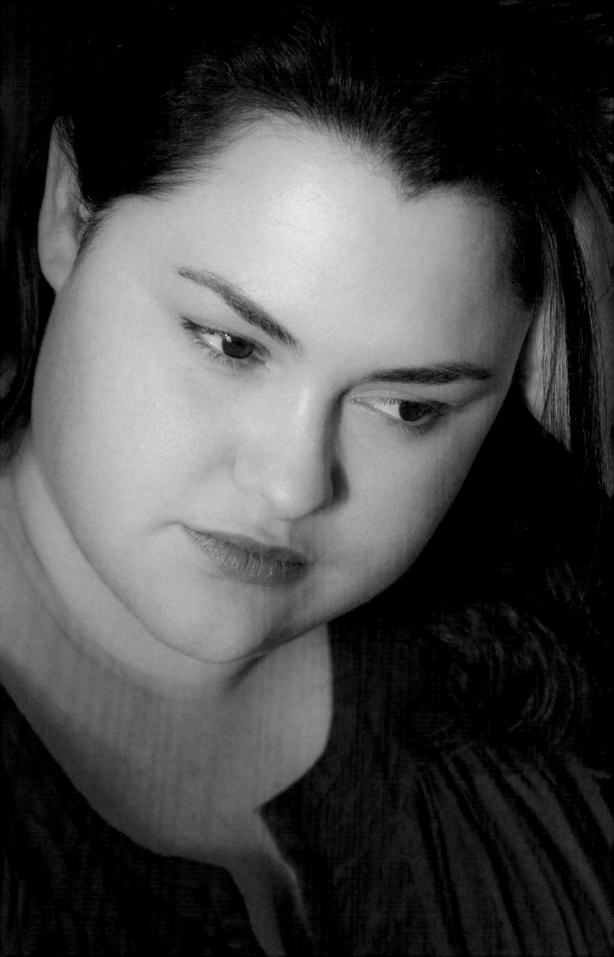

How many people get up in a rush, barely taking time to gulp down a coffee, and then eat a muffin or pastry at 10 a.m.? This often results in a drop in blood sugar around lunchtime, making them feel inordinately hungry. Too big a lunch makes us sleepy early in the afternoon. We often eat too much dinner too late, which is not at all good for sleep … especially if we add a small late-night snack in front of the TV. These late meals spoil our morning appetite, and the vicious cycle starts all over again. Water consumption is often overlooked. Many people drink sugary juices, milk, tea, coffee, alcohol, and salty soups, forgetting that these drinks are never as effective as water for staying hydrated.

Breakfast should include proteins (yogurt, eggs, cheese, nuts) and whole grains, as well as fruit. If a snack is needed during the morning, it should be "healthy," without concentrated sugar and not too high in calories. The midday meal should not be too large. Dinner should be eaten at least four hours before bed, possibly with a light snack planned at the end of the evening, to avoid nocturnal reflux. Some people need to eat small meals interspersed with snacks, while others function very well on three meals a day.

Increasing daily water consumption may decrease the frequency of attacks. It's generally thought that women should drink two litres of water a day and men, three litres — this adds up to eight to twelve cups respectively, or almost a glass every hour! Obviously, it's important to drink water throughout the day and not to guzzle a litre of water or herbal tea before going to bed, which would very likely mean waking up more than once during the night to urinate.

Dietary triggers

Many patients, before seeing a doctor, carry out a virtual witch-hunt for dietary triggers. Armed with long lists from books or the Internet (and sometimes from very reliable sources), they try to eliminate dozens of foods from their diet, often without much success. So why is this? There seem to be two main reasons. First of all, several foods have been labelled as attack triggers, but it must be remembered that

A Plant Trigger: The Headache Tree

Who would have thought that a tree could cause headaches? This is however the case for a species of bay laurel, the Umbellularia californica. The leaves of this tree emit a strong smell that can cause migraine attacks, as well as cluster headache. How can this fact, observed for hundreds of years by American Indian tribes in California, be explained?

The substance responsible is umbellulone, and it acts by stimulating a protein in the membrane of sensory neurons. This protein, TRPA1, has two main effects: vasodilation and the release of peptides associated with the calcitonin gene (CGRP). As we saw in Chapter 3, neurogenic inflammation, stimulated by CGRP, is one of the main mechanisms in a migraine attack. This story is a good illustration of how molecular science now makes it possible to understand formerly unexplained phenomena.

most of these foods are actually harmful to only a small percentage of the population. Only three foods have been formally tested: ice-cold products (ice water, ice, ice cream), wine, and chocolate, which seems to have been wrongly blamed (see Box on page 121)!

Migraine attacks are not exclusively associated with dietary triggers, so there may be many coincidences, especially with foods eaten regularly. If you eat bread every day, the fact you ate some on the day of a migraine attack doesn't necessarily mean it caused your attack. If you have very frequent migraines, the hunt for triggers can become exhausting and will probably not be very productive. Obviously, if you eat kiwis only rarely, your migraines are infrequent, and every time you eat kiwis you have a migraine, the association seems more likely. It must also be remembered that, according to the principle of the combination of triggers, a food may be a trigger during a risky period (for example, the menstrual period) and not the rest of the time. Some foods are suggested as triggers based on a chemical explanation (Figure 44). If you want to try to avoid triggers, begin with the most common. If you have a doubt about a specific food, use a diary to check your theory before changing your diet permanently.

Coffee: treatment or trigger?

Another apparent paradox in the world of migraines concerns caffeine. There's good reason to be puzzled, since caffeine is presented as both treatment and trigger. In fact, both claims are true. Caffeine is found in several combination painkillers used in

Five Pieces of Advice on Sleep to Reduce Migraines

1. Maintain a regular sleep schedule of seven to eight hours of sleep a night.
2. Stop reading, watching TV, or looking at a screen in bed.
3. Use a visualization technique to make it easier to fall asleep.
4. Have your evening meal four or more hours before going to bed and don't drink anything less than two hours before bed.
5. Stop taking afternoon naps.

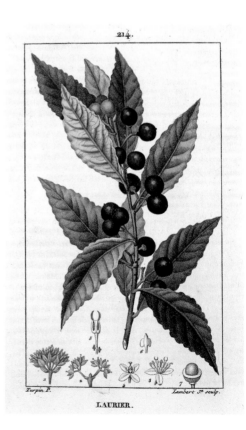

LAURIER.

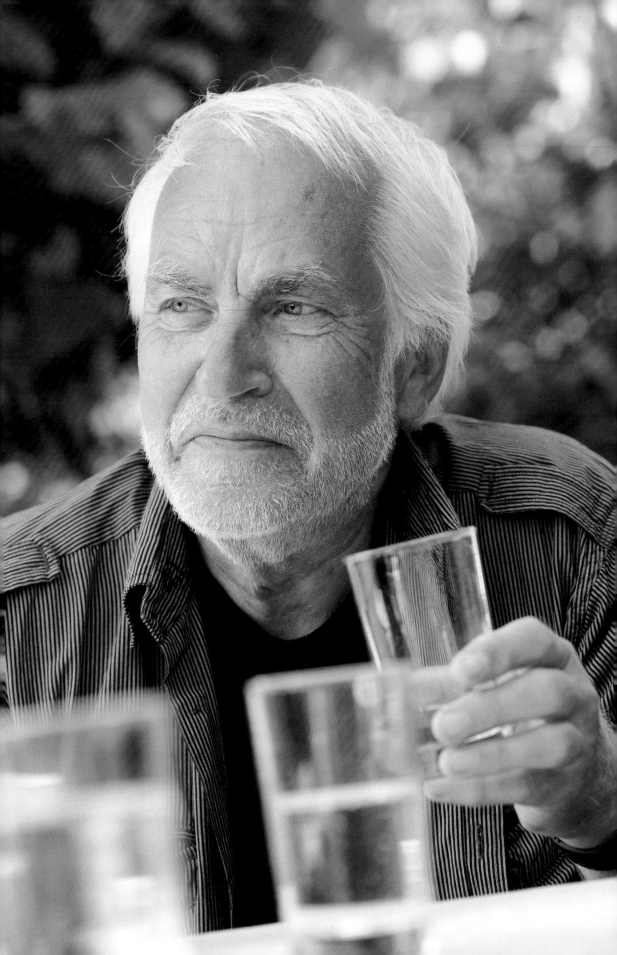

acute treatments (see Chapter 7). Caffeine has a definite stimulant effect; it heightens alertness, respiratory function, and muscle contraction. Many studies have shown a positive effect on athletic performance. Caffeine also has antidepressant and neuroprotective effects. If it's consumed regularly, however, its effect wears off, as the brain becomes accustomed to its biological actions. As soon as blood concentration of caffeine decreases, withdrawal may trigger an attack. Regular intake of caffeine is a factor in migraine chronification. It's also associated with chronic fatigue syndrome. As a result, caffeine may be considered an auxiliary treatment for migraine attacks, especially in people who don't consume it regularly. Stopping drinking coffee should be part of the treatment plan in cases of chronic migraine, especially if medication overuse is a problem.

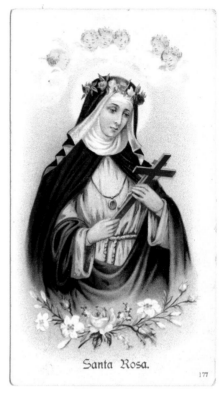

Santa Rosa.

↖ Perfection is not always possible.

WEIGHT LOSS ADVICE 101

PREPARATION	Keep a detailed food diary, for a month, for example.
	Calculate your Body Mass Index (BMI).
	Become aware of the reasons for your food habits.
	Set a realistic objective. Avoid miracle diets.
	Consult a dietician.
BASIC ADVICE	Eat at fixed times; don't skip meals.
	Eat slowly.
	Drink more water, less juice; eliminate soft drinks.
	Increase fibre intake, avoid foods high in sugar and fat.
	Eat healthy snacks, but beware of nibbling.
	Try new recipes and spend time cooking.
	Serve smaller portions; take time to taste your food.

FIGURE 43

Chocolate Doesn't Trigger Migraines!

Fewer than 5 percent of migraineurs say they are sensitive to chocolate. It even looks like chocolate doesn't trigger migraine, but that instead migraine actually triggers a craving for chocolate in the prodrome stage. Among sixty-three migraine sufferers enrolled in a study, 17 percent said chocolate was a trigger. The participants had to follow a tyramine-free diet for two weeks, and then eat a bar of chocolate or carob (tested together, since they taste identical). This test was repeated several times. There was no difference in the triggering of migraines between the two groups. That should reassure chocoholics!

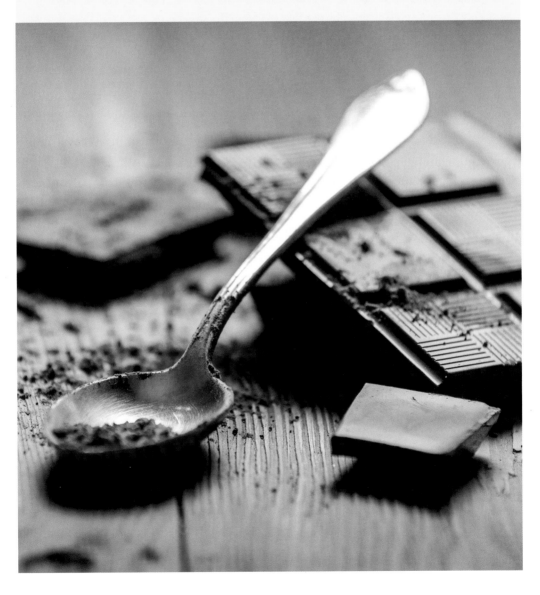

Food intolerances

Lactose-free and gluten-free diets are very fashionable, with many books having been published on this topic. Very often, migraine is mentioned among the problems that might be solved by a particular diet. It must be remembered that migraine is very common and is therefore a prime advertising target. But how true is this? Can migraines be cured if you quit consuming lactose, gluten, or meat protein?

Gluten is a molecule found in the grains commonly consumed in our societies. Celiac disease is a severe gluten intolerance caused by the production of antibodies that destroy the intestinal lining. Gluten intolerance is a less pronounced form. The antibodies typical of celiac disease are not present, but the symptoms reported by patients go away with a gluten-free diet and recur when gluten consumption resumes. A few studies associate gluten intolerance with migraines, but aside from anecdotes, there's no proof that a gluten-free diet can improve migraines.

EMOTIONAL FACTORS AND STRESS

Is stress really a migraine trigger? A very large number of migraineurs would no doubt answer yes to this question (Figure 40). It seems however that a reduction in stress is a more powerful trigger than chronic stress per se. The onset of migraines when stress levels decline may be caused by a drop in blood cortisol, in somewhat the same way that a decrease in estrogen triggers menstrual migraines. Determining the actual role of stress in a specific person's migraines is very difficult. Some healthcare professionals tend to blame stress alone to explain migraines, but this is going too far. Conversely, some migraine sufferers vigorously deny the impact of emotions on their attacks, which is sometimes unrealistic.

DIETARY CHEMICAL SUBSTANCES TRIGGERING MIGRAINES

CHEMICAL SUBSTANCE	FOOD
Aspartame	Colas and Other Diet Products
Monosodium Glutamate	Chinese Food, Soya Sauce
Histamine	Fermented Products
Nitrites	Processed Meats, Wieners
Sulfites	Wine, Dried Fruit
Tannins	Wine
Tyramine, Phenylethylamine	Aged Cheeses, Chocolate, Nuts, Citrus Fruit, Vinegar, Leftovers

FIGURE 44

Psychosomatic theories

In Chapter 2, we summarized the theories according to which migraine might be mainly psychosomatic. Because of these theories, many migraineurs have been stigmatized and almost accused of using their migraines to manipulate those around them. We've explained in this book that a migraine attack is a genuine neurological phenomenon whose mechanisms are increasingly understood. Biological, genetic, molecular, and pharmacological discoveries have allowed migraine sufferers to cast off the psychosomatic label that they had often been given up to the 1980s.

However, science evolves in pendulum-like movements, and just because an outmoded hypothesis has been relegated to the back of the drawer doesn't mean it has no value. Understanding the biological mechanisms of migraines is very important, but equally crucial is recognizing the influence of psychological and social factors on the brain.

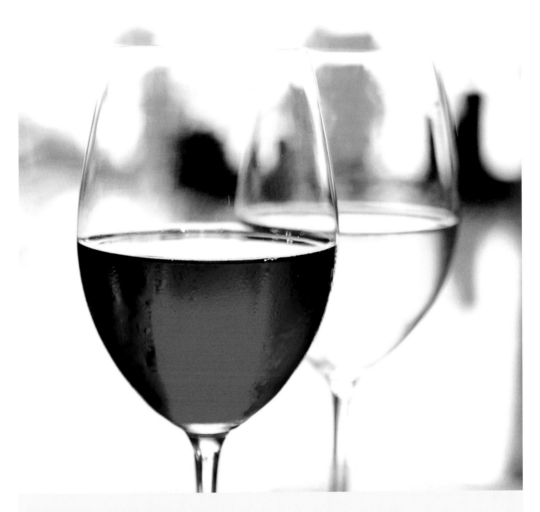

Alcohol and Migraine

To the regret of those who can no longer take part in champagne, beer, or wine toasts at various everyday celebrations, one of the best known food triggers is definitely alcohol. Between 17 and 76 percent of migraine sufferers describe a negative effect from alcohol in general. Several components in alcoholic beverages can affect the brain, including sulfites and tannins, found especially in red wine. Surprisingly, some people tolerate one kind of alcohol very well, but not another: there are those who can't even take a sip from a champagne glass, while others are only sensitive to craft beer. The role of genetics in these specific sensitivities may be speculated on, but knowledge on this subject is still limited.

Let's take an example from another medical field. In the 1960s, according to the tenets of psychoneuroimmunology, the idea was accepted that people convinced they were going to get better could activate their immune systems and, by so doing, cure themselves. This reassuring "mental force," to use the familiar expression, was very favourably received by the public. The importance of psychological factors is still recognized, although patient support does not replace chemotherapy.

It's therefore surprising to realize that many migraine sufferers are annoyed when links between their migraines and their psychological state are mentioned. In some cases, chronic migraine is associated with an uncontrollable stressful situation that has persisted for several years: a parent being cared for, marital problems, financial instability, a hostile workplace, unresolved post-traumatic stress. It isn't always possible to resolve these conflicts, change jobs, cure those around us, or control nightmares, but it may be helpful to get the support and guidance of a psychologist to work on perceptions of these situations and find ways of coping with them in everyday life. In some cases there are tough choices to be made and talking to a neutral professional can really clarify a person's thinking process.

Stress management tools, and managing schedules and energy
There never seems to be enough time; it's rare to find people who don't describe themselves as "overwhelmed." In our daily rat race, it sometimes seems impossible to set priorities. Faced with a pile-up of things to do, shorter and shorter nights, and increasing responsibilities, migraineurs can very easily fall prey to a storm of attacks. This can easily trigger a vicious cycle, since the attacks slow down functioning and force sufferers to put things off until later, increasing daily stress even more. No one is born with a doctorate in time management. In some cases, it's enough to apply a few pieces of advice to reset the clocks and regain control (see Box below). But sometimes in-depth work is needed, and professional help (from an occupational therapist or psychologist) may prove useful. Migraine may force us to take life more slowly, and sometimes quality of life will be enhanced if we accept some compromises in our everyday routines. People often emphasize the fact that medications are not natural, but nor is it natural to sleep five hours a night or to spend fifteen hours a day looking at screens.

Seven Points to Work on to Improve Time Management

1. Aim to work at a regular pace and not in spurts of hyperactivity leading to exhaustion.
2. Divide the work into concrete stages and set up a realistic timeline.
3. Decide to work more slowly and include rest periods.
4. Learn to say no and listen to yourself instead of wanting to please other people.
5. Learn to recognize warning signs when you're overwhelmed.
6. Use stress management techniques.
7. Use "pressure valves" to relax, including enjoyable activities.

BIOFEEDBACK

This therapeutic technique may be used for various painful medical conditions or for anxiety disorders. It involves observing the body's reactions to stress so as to learn to lower the tension level, with the aim of calming and stabilizing the body and brain activity. The symptoms of tension observed include the contraction of certain muscles (temporal, jaw, trapezius), heart rate, the temperature of the hands and feet, and respiration rate. Measuring devices can be used to detect signs of stress in the body. Subsequently, breathing or relaxation exercises are learned, and their effect on the symptoms of stress is observed. It may be very reassuring to note that, simply by controlling your breathing, you can lower arterial pressure and warm up your hands!

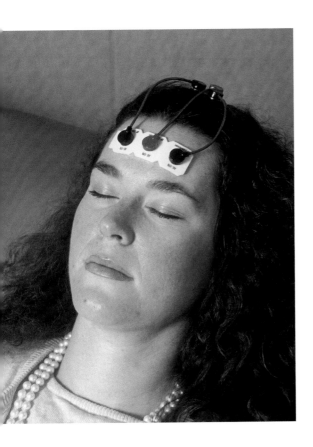

Biofeedback is a tested and effective technique for managing migraines, but learning it requires an investment in time and effort. The process takes weeks, sometimes months, and requires the help of a skilled therapist, usually a psychologist. The major advantage of biofeedback is the total absence of side effects and the ability to apply the acquired techniques in many situations. Children and teenagers are very sensitive to the effect of biofeedback. The problem is that it's not always easy to find a certified professional. A more recent form of therapy, neurofeedback, analyses brain activity using electrodes placed on the skull. Neurofeedback therapists report this to be effective in controlling migraines, but there are few studies on the topic.

MEDITATION AND RELAXATION TECHNIQUES

Meditation is a term that covers many Eastern and Western concepts, including prayer, philosophical reflection, breathing exercises, or a daily walk. The word "meditation" is derived from the name of Melete, the muse of meditation and exercise in Greek mythology. All meditation techniques have to be practised regularly to be effective. The approach known as "mindfulness" has been developed by Jon Kabat-Zinn, a researcher at the Massachusetts Institute of Technology, with the goal of better managing stress and chronic pain. The original technique is based on an eight-week program. A few studies on meditation for relieving migraine exist, but this is a field that's still developing.

PSYCHOTHERAPY

Using the services of a psychologist must be considered if a mental health problem influences migraines. However,

Amelia, 32

In her work as a secretary, Amelia is constantly in demand. She finds it hard to drink enough water, because when she drinks she has to leave her desk often to go to the washroom. In the evening she drinks herbal tea to make up for it, but spends the night going to the toilet. What's more, in the morning it's such a mad dash with her two daughters that she doesn't have time to eat breakfast. Nor does she have time to exercise....

After a few painful attacks, Amelia took herself in hand. She started taking a water bottle to work and allowed herself time to go to the washroom. In the morning she has a glass of water and a protein bar. She keeps Tuesday evenings free for a dance class, and in return her partner spends Thursday evenings with his friends. She's still tired sometimes, but the attacks are farther apart, and she has learned not to neglect herself!

psychotherapy can also be used to manage chronic pain and its impacts on mood. In such cases, the cognitive-behavioural approach may focus on negative thoughts, like feelings of guilt and worthlessness, and replace them with more positive thoughts. Acceptance and engagement therapy is one of the therapies sometimes used to manage chronic pain. The therapist may also offer helpful support and a space for a neutral discussion of the difficulties being experienced. Patients are often fearful of the idea of beginning therapy and wonder how much time they'll have to devote to it, how much it will cost, and how their decision will be perceived by those around them. This is however an important decision that may lead to a genuine improvement in quality of life.

EXERCISE AND YOGA

There are countless benefits to physical activity, but it can sometimes seem impossible to find room for two hours of exercise in a busy week. Although the Canadian guidelines recommend that adults get thirty minutes of cardiovascular activity per day, fewer than 15 percent of adult Canadians follow these recommendations.

Regular exercise keeps the body toned and increases its resistance to daily stressors. For someone in good shape, climbing stairs, carrying packages, and walking for twenty minutes is not really exertion or stress. But for someone who is used to sitting a lot or who is not in shape, these small everyday activities are an effort ... and possibly a migraine trigger. Exercise is also an excellent way to get rid of stress and keep sleep regular. It's been said a thousand times, but let's say it again: a healthy mind in a healthy body. Too often, doctors tend not to bother giving advice on physical activity, taking it for granted that their patients won't follow it. Yet exercise is as effective as many medications and should in fact be prescribed as seriously as any pill (see Box on page 127).

Yoga has been studied in relation to migraine management. Evidence of a positive effect on the frequency of attacks actually does exist. Yoga is not necessarily easy or safe, however. Some postures can be hard on the neck. Others require significant muscle strength, which some unfit people have lost. People who aren't in very good physical condition should therefore choose

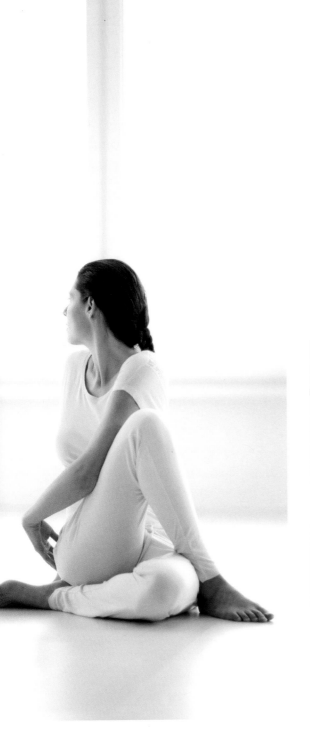

a beginners' class and let the instructor know their fitness status, or go directly to a therapeutic yoga instructor.

Migraineurs need to provide their brains with optimal operating conditions. Taking charge of yourself, looking after yourself, and taking care of your body should be looked on as a gift you give yourself and not as a punishment you inflict. Some patients miss being able to stay out late, drink alcohol, eat fatty foods, watch TV before going to bed, etc. This says a lot about our society of abundance, leisure activities, and sedentary behaviour, where we're perfectly free to do ourselves harm. In any event, managing lifestyle habits is undeniably the first stage in treating migraines.

Advice for Choosing a Physical Activity

1. It will be hard at first. Expect to persevere for at least two months.
2. Keep a diary of your sessions.
3. Choose an activity adapted to your abilities and one that fits easily into your schedule.
4. Keep an open mind; try something new that interests you.
5. Exercise with someone or in a group.
6. Aim for regularity rather than intensity.
7. If physical activity triggers your attacks, get professional help to adapt your practice.
8. Become aware of the benefits of exercise. And above all, pat yourself on the back!

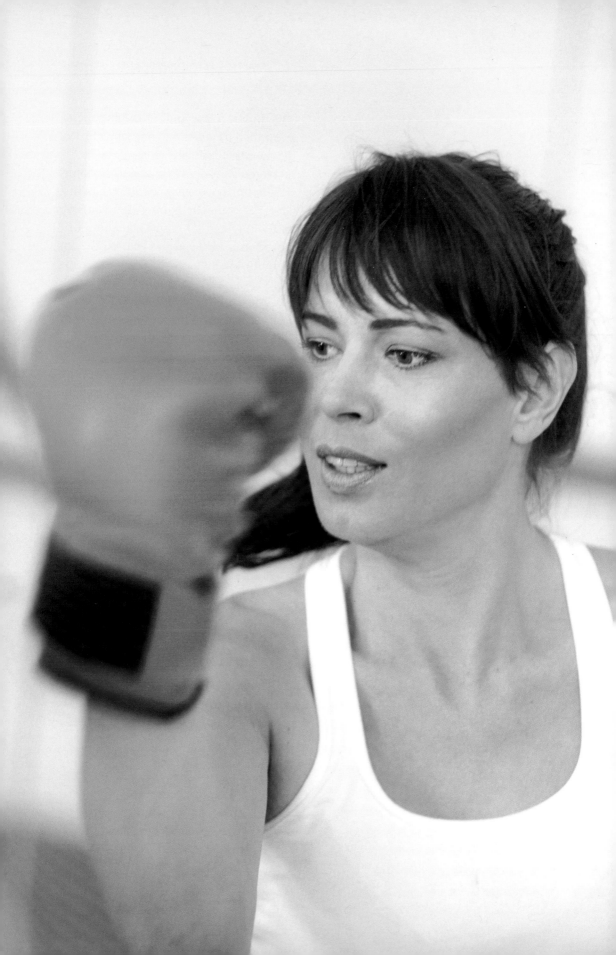

CHAPTER 7

Treating the Attack

I had a terrible migraine; I was not thinking anymore,
I was not living, I was indifferent to everything.

— George Sand, *Story of My Life*

You were dreading it, you felt it coming on, and now you know: the attack has started. The first symptoms appear. If you suffer from severe attacks and you don't have an acute treatment handy, this means you're in for a very bad day. What can you do to avoid ending up in bed nauseated, or sitting in front of your computer, looking pale and working in slow motion? How can you avoid cancelling your evening with friends? And above all, how can you avoid winding up in the emergency room?

Many migraineurs will never need to see a doctor; their attacks will remain infrequent and be easy to treat with over-the-counter medications. But if you've tried these drugs, have sought advice from the pharmacist, and in spite of everything are still unable to function because of your attacks, you need to get more appropriate treatment, often by prescription. Several attempts are sometimes necessary to find the option that suits you (see Box on page 131). An ineffective treatment must be abandoned, while a reliable and tolerated treatment will be adopted for the long term.

THE GOAL OF ACUTE TREATMENT

The goal of an acute treatment is a return to normal activities, ideally without having to spend time in bed. Of course, in the case of severe attacks, you may have to lie down for a while to stop the attack completely, but if you have to spend the afternoon lying down because of your migraine, you might want to look for a new acute treatment. Patients' expectations for acute treatments have been studied. The results of these studies indicate that the treatment should not only relieve the headache, but also the related migraine symptoms, like light intolerance and nausea. The side effects should not prevent a return to normal activities. The effect should be reliable and reproducible from one attack to another.

AVAILABLE TREATMENTS

Several drug classes are available to interrupt a migraine attack. The main drugs used are acetaminophen, anti-inflammatories,

Six Basic Concepts in the Choice of an Acute Treatment

1. The goal of an acute treatment is to make a return to normal activities possible within two hours after the treatment is taken.
2. There is no "better treatment" for migraine attacks. Everyone reacts differently to different molecules.
3. The only way to find an effective and tolerated treatment is to try different ones and note the success of each strategy.
4. Whichever treatment is used, taking it quickly, at the beginning of the attack, increases its chances of success.
5. If the attacks are not well controlled by one medication, combinations must be tried.
6. Some migraine sufferers have attacks of varying intensity and therefore need different combinations adapted to each situation.

triptans, and rye ergot derivatives. The history of all of these drugs is rooted in plant-based medicinal treatment. Anti-nausea drugs are often taken in conjunction with other treatments if the nausea is severe. Opiates, or narcotics, should generally be avoided in treating migraine; this will be discussed again later.

ACETAMINOPHEN AND COMBINATION PAINKILLERS

This simple or first-level painkiller is easy to obtain and sometimes effective ... but not very often. In Canada and the United States, several acetaminophen, caffeine, and codeine combinations exist. These combinations may be more effective than acetaminophen alone, but come with a higher risk of medication-overuse headache.

NON-STEROIDAL ANTI-INFLAMMATORIES OR NSAIDS

These anti-inflammatories are called "non-steroidal," to distinguish them from cortisone, which is one of the steroids and also has anti-inflammatory properties. Migraine attacks are caused by neurogenic inflammation triggered by the brain, as we saw in Chapter 3. It's therefore not surprising that anti-inflammatories are useful for interrupting a migraine attack. There are several kinds of anti-inflammatories, the most common being aspirin and ibuprofen (Figure 45). Naproxen is an NSAID often prescribed to relieve migraines and has the advantage of being long-lasting. Nonetheless, some patients would still rather take ibuprofen in Liqui-Gel form; it has a shorter duration of drug action, but takes effect more quickly. A recent form, diclofenac potassium powder (Cambia), is very rapidly absorbed. The various NSAIDs

COMMON ACUTE TREATMENTS: ANTI-INFLAMMATORIES

NSAID	Dosage Available in Canada	Dosage Recommended for Migraine	Available Forms	Comments
IBUPROFEN* (ADVIL, MOTRIN)	200-400 mg	400 mg	Oral: Tablets and Liqui-Gel	Available without prescription.
NAPROXEN* (NAPROSYN, ANAPROX)	200 mg Over the counter 125, 250, 375, 500 mg Sodic 550 mg	500 to 825 mg	Oral: Tablet Oral: Liquid Suspension Suppository	Long half-life. The sodic form is absorbed more quickly.
ACETYLSALICYLIC ACID* (ASPIRIN)	80-325-500-650-975 mg	975 to 1000 mg	Oral: Tablet and Effervescent Tablet Suppository	Exists in combination with caffeine (ANACIN).
DICLOFENAC POTASSIUM* (VOLTAREN RAPID)	50 mg	50 mg	Oral: Tablet	
DICLOFENAC POTASSIUM* (CAMBIA)	50 mg	50 mg	Oral: Water-Soluble Powder	Very fast acting. Menthol and licorice flavour.
INDOMETHACIN (INDOCID)	25-50-100 mg	50 to 100 mg	Oral: Capsule Suppository	Occasionally poorly tolerated but sometimes very effective.
KETOROLAC** (TORADOL)	10 or 30 mg vial	30 mg	Injectable Intramuscular	Practical for violent attacks. Injection technique has to be taught.

* Recommended in the Canadian acute migraine treatment guidelines.
** Recommended for treating migraine attacks in the emergency room, but can be used at home.

FIGURE 45

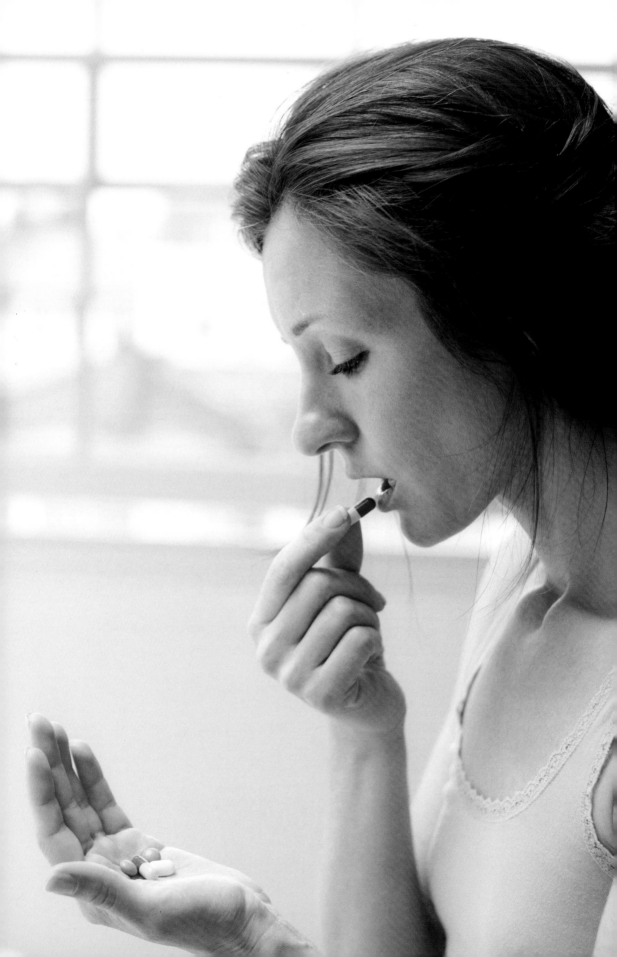

The History of Triptans

In the Middle Ages, rye bread was part of the normal diet of monks and peasants. In rainy weather, rye is attacked by the *Claviceps purpurea* fungus, also known as rye ergot. "Ergot" comes from the Old French "argot," meaning "cock's spur," which the fungus on a rye stalk vaguely resembles. Harvested with the grain, it was ground and incorporated into the flour. But it contained a substance later known as ergotamine that stimulates the brain's serotonin receptors and the arteries in the human brain. Eating contaminated rye bread can have disastrous consequences, including hallucinations and extremely painful gangrene: St. Anthony's fire or holy fire. To find a cure, those with the disease used to undertake a pilgrimage to pray to St. Anthony. This journey was often viewed as miraculous, for when they stopped eating the bread poisoned with rye ergot, their blood circulation returned to normal and the gangrene disappeared.

After much observation, the effects of Claviceps purpurea on the arteries were eventually understood, and in the nineteenth century uterine hemorrhaging began to be treated using a paste of ground rye ergot to constrict the uterine arteries.

Migraine had already long been associated with dilation of the arteries. At some point, someone had the idea of using *Claviceps purpurea* to treat it. And thus was born ergotamine, a medical treatment derived from the *Claviceps purpurea* fungus.

Science progressed, and in the 1950s serotonin receptors were discovered. The word "serotonin" reflects its vasoconstrictive properties: *sero*, found in the serum or blood, and *tonin*, increasing vascular tonus. Serotonin's neurological properties, including its role in mood management, would be discovered much later. Once it had been synthesized in a laboratory, sumatriptan, a selective serotonin agonist whose vascular effects are less powerful than those of ergotamine, came onto the market in 1980. This was truly a revolution. Thousands of migraine sufferers discovered they could stop their attacks without spending days in bed.

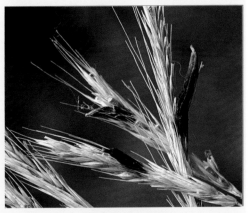

↖ Rye ergot: *Claviceps purpurea.*

have different chemical structures, which is why the effects of each type vary from person to person. NSAIDs may cause heartburn. It's sometimes recommended that they be taken with a little food, not always possible during an attack.

Some people can't use anti-inflammatories. People with inflammatory diseases of the intestine (ulcerative colitis, Crohn's disease), uncontrolled high blood pressure, kidney failure, active stomach ulcers, or allergies must not take these drugs.

TRIPTANS

Triptans have literally revolutionized the world of migraine (see Box on previous page). The prescription of an appropriate triptan really can change a migraine patient's life.

Triptans are designed to treat migraines. They're not painkillers: it's useless to take them for backache or toothache! They act specifically on the serotonin receptors in the brain by stimulating them. We still don't know exactly why this action on the serotonin system has the effect of interrupting a migraine attack. In the brain, serotonin receptors are located in the cerebral arteries, in the brain stem, and throughout the cortex. It's possible that triptans act in several different ways.

Since sumatriptan appeared, six other triptans have come onto the market (Figure 48). Most of them now have generic equivalents. Their effectiveness is believed to be higher than that of acetaminophen (Figure 46). Despite this, only 10 to 20 percent of people with migraine claim to use them. Why? The optimal use of triptans hinges on several factors (see box on page 135).

Although triptans are very effective for the majority of migraineurs, they are not effective for everyone. Nearly 30 percent of the population is insensitive to their action. A genetic cause has been suggested to explain this statistic. However, before declaring someone to be triptan-insensitive, it's essential to try several, since the effectiveness of the various triptans varies from person to person. The main contra-indications are pregnancy (to be discussed with the doctor), poorly controlled high blood pressure, vascular diseases (coronary heart disease, stroke, artery failure in the legs) and, in some cases, intolerances. Allergies to triptans are very rare.

Concerns about triptans

Very often, triptans are perceived as dangerous, and their price is quite high compared to anti-inflammatories. This contributes to their image of being powerful and therefore dangerous. By stimulating the serotonin receptors, they cause a slight vasoconstriction of the arteries. For this reason, they can't be prescribed for people with poorly controlled high blood pressure, heart disease, or those who've had a stroke. Again, because of their action on serotonin receptors, triptans have been the object of a warning from the Food and Drug Administration (FDA) recommending they not be prescribed to people taking antidepressants, since these also stimulate the serotonin system. The stimulatory effect of the two drugs combined could result in serotonin syndrome, a potentially dangerous reaction in the organism. But the American Headache Society has reviewed all cases of serotonin syndrome in relation to triptans and has determined that the risk of developing this syndrome because of triptans is negligible. And let's not forget that these drugs have been taken safely by millions of people for more than twenty years.

Barriers to the Optimal Use of Triptans

1. Limited access to a prescription, especially for a patient without a family doctor.
2. Family doctors likely not adequately trained with regard to triptans.
3. Disproportionate fears of doctors, pharmacists, and the public concerning the risks of triptans.
4. Insufficient instructions given to patients, unproductive trials.
5. Insufficient number of refills on prescriptions.
6. Prohibitive cost, partial reimbursement by insurance companies.

GREATER SATISFACTION WITH TRIPTANS THAN WITH ACETAMINOPHEN

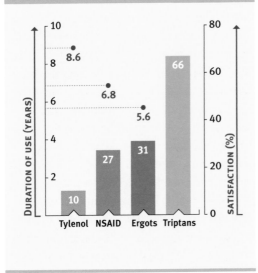

FIGURE 46   Diamond, *Am J Med*, 2005.

Triptan exhaustion

Triptan exhaustion is a phenomenon well known to doctors. Sometimes, without our knowing exactly why, a triptan that has been effective for many years becomes less reliable. First of all, it must be determined that this loss of effectiveness is not because of overuse. If a triptan is being taken more than ten days a month, this may be the problem, and withdrawal should be considered. But if overuse is not the problem, it could be exhaustion (not a recognized scientific term, but a word commonly used in practice). In this situation, the best thing to do is change the triptan. Sometimes, after a few months' pause, the "exhausted" triptan becomes effective again. To avoid exhaustion, some patients alternate two triptans (while still being careful about overuse), but we don't know if this technique is really effective.

RYE ERGOT DERIVATIVES

These drugs are the ancestors of triptans. Ergotamine (Cafergot) is now used very seldom in North America, but its use is quite common in Latin America. Dihydroergotamine (DHE) is, on the other hand, very useful, since it has the reputation of not causing medication-overuse headache. Some protocols including DHE in intravenous or subcutaneous form are used by headache clinics for withdrawal, or for chronic headaches that are difficult to control, as well as for *status migrainosus*. There is also an intranasal form of DHE, but absorption is less reliable and often triggers unpleasant dryness in the mucous membranes. A pump-inhaler form is being studied.

LATE TREATMENT LEADS TO FAILURE

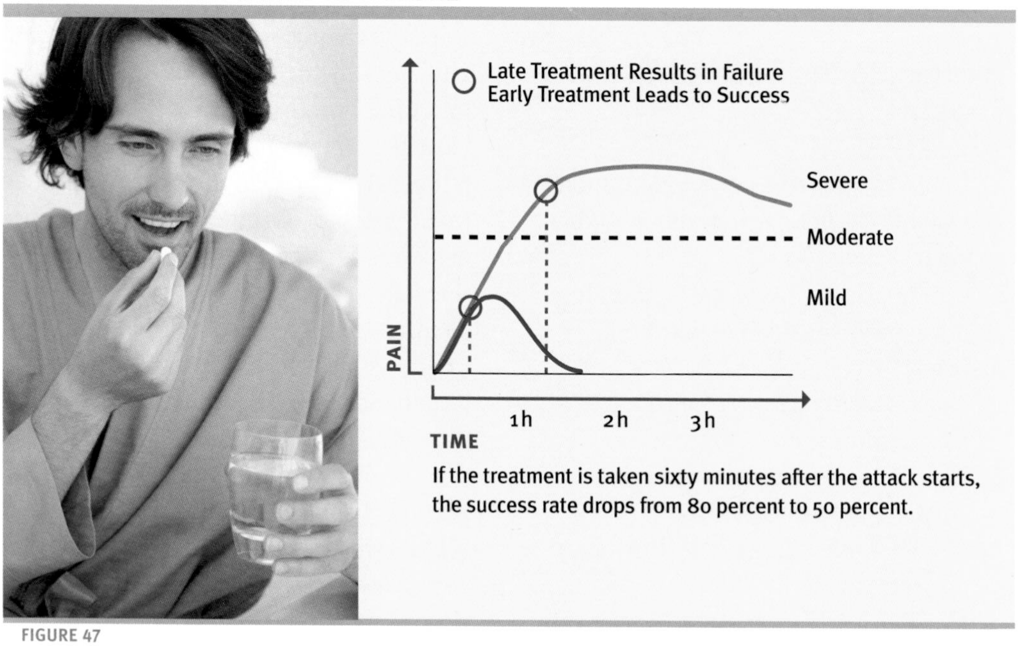

Late Treatment Results in Failure
Early Treatment Leads to Success

Severe

Moderate

Mild

PAIN

TIME

1 h   2 h   3 h

If the treatment is taken sixty minutes after the attack starts, the success rate drops from 80 percent to 50 percent.

FIGURE 47

ANTIEMETICS

Acute migraine treatment may include a drug to control nausea. Dimenhydrinate (Gravol) is the most common option. Some antidopaminergic antiemetics administered intravenously (metoclopramide, prochlorperazine, chlorpromazine) also have an anti-migraine action and are often used in emergency rooms. Sleepiness is a common side effect and adverse reactions like low blood pressure or dystonic symptoms are sometimes observed.

NARCOTICS: WHY THEY MUST BE AVOIDED

Narcotics, or opiates, include several molecules from the morphine family (Statex). The main forms in circulation are codeine, oxycodone, hydromorphone, and fentanyl. New formulations have appeared more recently, including buprenorphine, tramadol, and many others. These drugs used to be reserved for cancer-related pain and acute and post-operative pain. In the 1990s, based on advice from experts and not on scientific studies, narcotics were recommended for the treatment of chronic pain, like back and neck pain, as well as for fibromyalgia. Today, the narcotics market has exploded, as has addiction to prescription drugs, and the United States consumes 80 percent of the world's opiates. The medical community has been forced to realize that the chronic use of narcotics may have serious consequences: dependence, criminal use, hip fractures, and car accidents (Figure 50). But most important: even if patients treated with narcotics claim their pain has been somewhat relieved, their ability to function in daily life and their quality of life are usually not really any better. Chronic pain has been examined in detail in a number of books. Its management must be based on a holistic and comprehensive approach, and not just by prescribing narcotics.

ACUTE TREATMENTS: TRIPTANS

Triptan (In Order of Appearance on the Market)	Dosages Available in Canada	Forms Available in Canada	Comments The Response to a Triptan Varies Greatly from Person to Person.
IMITREX SUMATRIPTAN	25–50–100 mg 5–20 mg 6 mg	Tablet Nasal Spray Injectable	First triptan on the market. Preferred triptan in several studies. Some pregnancy data available.
ZOMIG ZOLMITRIPTAN	1 or 2.5 mg 1 or 2.5 mg 2.5 or 5 mg	Tablet Dissolving Tablet Nasal Spray	The nasal spray is a good option for violent attacks, but be prepared for an unpleasant taste.
MAXALT RIZATRIPTAN	5 or 10 mg 5 or 10 mg	Tablet Dissolving Tablet	Fast action. A few pediatric studies, but not approved by Health Canada for children.
AMERGE NARATRIPTAN	1 or 2.5 mg	Tablet	Very long duration of drug action. Longer onset of action. Fewer side effects.
RELPAX ELETRIPTAN	40 mg	Tablet	Less recurrence according to some studies.
AXERT ALMOTRIPTAN	6.25 mg 12.5 mg	Tablet	Authorized by Health Canada for those 12 and over. Fewer side effects.
FROVA FROVATRIPTAN	2.5 mg	Tablet	Very long-lasting. Slower to take effect. Fewer side effects.

All triptans are contra-indicated if vascular disease is a problem (infarctus, coronary disease, stroke, poorly controlled hypertension, etc.).

These medications are only available by prescription, and their safe and effective use must be discussed with a doctor. Most triptans are now available as generics.

FIGURE 48

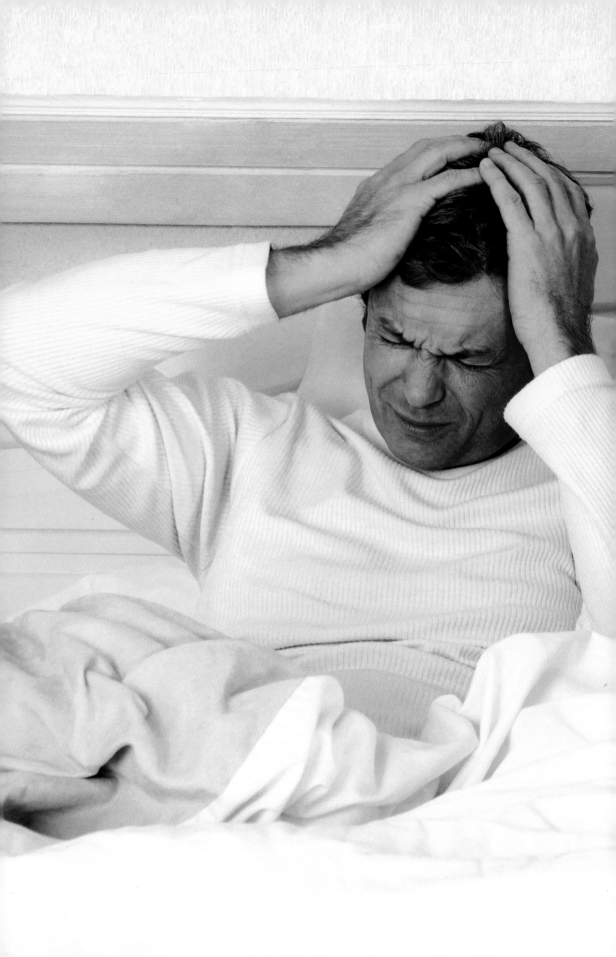

Narcotics are often prescribed to treat migraines, especially in the United States, where triptans are not always reimbursed by insurance companies. These medications have several disadvantages that lead most specialists in the headache field to avoid using them. Side effects such as apathy, constipation, and nausea may occur. However, the main problem is their very strong tendency to cause dependence and rebound or medication-overuse headache. Some authors suggest that taking narcotics on more than seven days a month may result in headache chronification. A renowned researcher in Michigan, Dr. Joel Saper, has managed a centre for refractory headaches for decades.

NARCOTICS: A RISKY OPTION

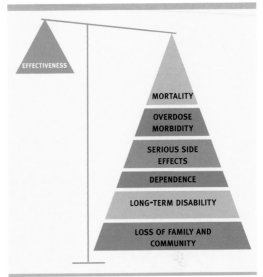

FIGURE 50   Adapted from Franklin, "Opioids for chronic non-cancer pain," *Neurology*, 2014.

ATTACK CHARACTERISTICS INFLUENCING TREATMENT CHOICE

Characteristic	Possibility	Result of Treatment Choice
TYPE OF ATTACK	One type only or several types	When there are several types of attack, it may be necessary to use several different combinations.
WARNING SIGNS	Presence of prodrome or aura	If you have warning signs, it's easy to treat the attack quickly. If the attack strikes without warning, it's more difficult.
SPEED OF PAIN ONSET	Slow or fast increase	An attack that occurs quickly is harder to control.
DIGESTIVE SYMPTOMS	Presence of nausea or vomiting	These symptoms indicate that drugs taken orally will likely not work.
ONSET TIMING	Attacks that occur at night or on waking	An already advanced attack present on waking makes management more difficult. "Fast-acting" options should be considered.
USUAL LENGTH OF ATTACK	Pain tends to come back, evidence of relapse	Long-lasting attacks are very frustrating. Adding long-lasting anti-inflammatories may prevent recurrence.

FIGURE 49

You Have to Treat the Headache in Time

It's a classic situation. Let's say you're at work. You had a bad night, and maybe you didn't have time to eat lunch. A slight pain in the temple appears — the first sign. According to your lengthy (too lengthy) experience, an hour or two from now the pain will be more intense, you'll no longer be able to concentrate on your work, and between now and the end of the day, you'll feel sick to your stomach. The most reasonable thing to do would be to take a pill. But already you hear a little voice saying, "Are you really sure this is a migraine? Maybe it will go away by itself…. What about having a small glass of water…. Anyway, you've left your Zomig in the car and surely you're not really going to waste time going to get it…. And remember, your neighbour told you that these drugs are strong and might make you dependent…. Last time, you were exhausted after taking one, so wait a while…." All of these arguments win out over your motivation. Two glasses of water later, the pain is stronger. Is there still time to treat it?

Initially convinced of the effectiveness of narcotics, he prescribed them to a great many otherwise refractory patients. In 2008, he published several articles describing his experience and summarizing his recommendations for migraine management. According to him, even with close multidisciplinary monitoring (follow-up that most doctors are not able to offer), fewer than 10 percent of patients really benefit from taking narcotics for their chronic headaches.

We don't have any totally effective treatments for migraines. The temptation of narcotics very often appeals to people living with the disease. In some cases, they may be very sporadically useful, as a treatment of last resort to avoid a trip to emergency for an exceptionally severe attack. It must be emphasized that, in the vast majority of cases, narcotics, despite an initial benefit, can harm the patient and lead to disastrous and hard-to-control consequences. The decision to use narcotics for a chronic refractory headache should be taken by a doctor experienced in this specific field of medicine and able to offer appropriate follow-up.

OTHER TECHNIQUES: OPTIMIZING TREATMENT

As we saw in Chapter 2, there has been no lack of eccentric treatments in the history of migraine. From rose-perfumed baths to our grandmothers' potato slices, to menthol gels, cooling caps, and acupressure point massage, options abound. It's impossible to describe all of these techniques, which for the most part have not been scientifically proven in any case. Remember that it's essential to be sure that the planned treatment is safe and, if it isn't effective, it should be stopped. Remember as well that the placebo effect of a treatment may actually interrupt a migraine attack, which is no small thing.

FACTORS TO CONSIDER: HOW WOULD YOU DESCRIBE YOUR ATTACKS?

The usual pattern of your attacks is one of the more important factors to consider

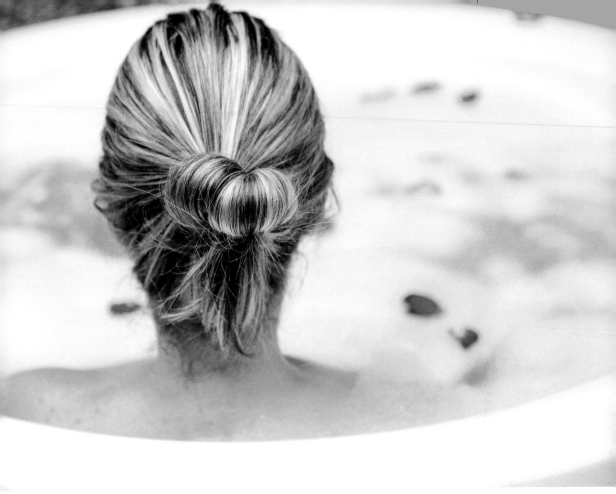

in choosing your acute treatment. Do you have several types of attacks or just one? The elements to note are summarized in the table of characteristics on page 139 (Figure 49).

FAST-ACTING OPTIONS

Some migraine sufferers have violent attacks that may be accompanied by vomiting and a total inability to function. These attacks can last several days if they are not controlled right from the start. During a migraine attack, the stomach often works more slowly than usual — this is called migraine gastroparesis, or weak stomach — preventing the absorption of drugs even when there is no nausea as yet. If the stomach is weak, other ways must be found to take the medications. There are several options.

Dissolving or sublingual forms (under the tongue)

The substances available in this form are not actually absorbed more quickly than ordinary tablets, but they have the advantage of not requiring a glass of water. Saliva is enough to dissolve them for you to swallow them. However, they sometimes have a strong taste that some patients don't like.

Suppositories

They are usually not very popular, as insertion into the rectum seems to be difficult for some people. This is nonetheless an option that should not be overlooked. The rectum is irrigated by veins that absorb the medication quickly, which means that an intrarectal drug is almost as fast-acting as

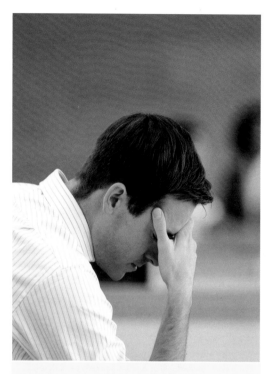

A Successful Treatment

Since being prepared is half the battle,
I lose nothing by taking precautions.
MIGUEL DE CERVANTES

You're at work after a very short night. The last few weeks have been exhausting. This morning, you didn't have time for breakfast. Around 10 o'clock, you feel pressure in your right temple: the first sign of migraine. Action ... reaction! In your desk drawer you have your medication, and you have a bottle of water with you. You take your treatment right away and in addition you take a few minutes to breathe. Half an hour later, the pain is gone. You can start your meeting with confidence ... and plan to go to bed early tonight!

an intravenous one! When you use a suppository, you must be sure to insert it fully. In theory, once it's placed beyond the anal sphincter, the rectal ampulla draw it in and prevent it from falling out. Some patients have trouble using suppositories, as they're afraid to insert them deeply enough. Explanation is sometimes necessary to make sure they are used correctly.

Intranasal sprays

This kind of spray is often very useful. The medication is sprayed into the nose and absorbed by the nasal mucosa. It sometimes takes a bit of experience to coordinate the spraying and inhaling properly, but once the technique has been learned, it's very useful. Since the medication is rapidly absorbed, the level in the blood is a little higher and side effects can be more pronounced. Some of the product is swallowed, which is normal, but the taste is sometimes unpleasant. Taking a small sip of juice helps it all go down.

Injections

Few people like the idea of having to inject themselves with drugs. But, in some cases, it's an option that saves the day. There are several kinds of injectable medications. Some require preparing the syringe at home — in other words you have to learn to draw the product out of the vial and then inject yourself with a standard syringe. This requires training supervised by a nurse. Other products are available in auto-injectors that look a little like an EpiPen and are easier to use. The injectable options have the advantage of speed, but side effects are sometimes more pronounced than for tablets. It may however be preferable to live with a few side effects instead of a really bad attack.

COMBINATIONS

Patients often worry about taking several medications at the same time to treat an attack. Once again, this natural distrust may be harmful, since some violent migraine attacks cannot be controlled with a single drug. NSAIDs and triptans have different action mechanisms and, in some cases, they have to be combined right at the beginning of the attack to be successful. In other situations, if the nausea is severe, an anti-nausea drug must be included in the acute treatment.

WHEN SHOULD I TAKE MY MEDICATION?

The decision to take an acute treatment at the right time is often more complex than it appears.

From a practical point of view, the effectiveness of treatments, especially triptans, is greatest when they are taken before the attack has advanced to the stage of severe pain or allodynia (Figure 47). Once the neurons have become hypersensitive and inflamed, triptans are less effective. In practice, this means that if allodynia or cutaneous hypersensitivity has set in, the likelihood of controlling your attack is lessened.

Many studies have shown that a migraine attack is easier to control if it's responded to quickly. Patients sometimes say: "The drug the doctor gave me may be almost miraculous, but I have to take it at the beginning of my attack; otherwise it's too late, the attack progresses, and nothing works." Why, then, do migraineurs put off taking their acute treatments for so long? This almost universal behaviour makes life difficult for doctors and patients. Here are a few reasons, along with some suggested solutions for a better outcome.

A FEW THOUGHTS ABOUT ACUTE TREATMENTS

I DON'T HAVE MY PILLS WITH ME

If you don't have attacks very often, you're more likely to forget to replenish your drug supplies. But it's really useful to carry your pills with you everywhere: in your purse, in your car, at work, etc. That way, no delay, no excuses ... and better control.

THE ATTACK WILL GO AWAY BY ITSELF

All migraine sufferers are normal and in perfect health ... until their next attack. The tendency toward wilful blindness is very widespread. Sufferers very often they know what will happen, but try to convince themselves of the contrary. The solution: observation using a diary. How often do your attacks really go away by themselves? If some headaches don't get worse, so much the better, but in that case try to identify signs that will tell you when a real attack is starting. People are all different and experience their attacks personally. You're the only one who can observe what you feel.

TYLENOL WILL HELP ME

It's true that some migraine attacks are treated with Tylenol, but according to scientific studies, they are not the majority. If the "take Tylenol" stage doesn't work, stop taking it. It won't help control the attack, and taking acetaminophen regularly can contribute to the rebound effect.

I GET SIDE EFFECTS FROM MY ACUTE TREATMENTS

This is entirely possible. NSAIDS may cause heartburn. Triptans sometimes cause nausea, fatigue, and even a tightness in the chest or jaw that can be worrying. If you're not tolerating your medications well, discuss them with your doctor. Another option should be tried. Everyone is different.

THE TREATMENTS ARE EXPENSIVE AND MY INSURANCE DOESN'T COVER THEM

This is a genuine problem. Triptans are expensive molecules, even in their generic forms. Insurance often covers a good portion of the cost, but the difference can be significant on a tight budget. Check with your pharmacist or doctor to see if less expensive options are available. And if you are limited, get the most out of your medications: if you delay taking them you waste your investment. Remember, too, that a lost workday costs money.

I'M AFRAID OF TAKING MEDICINES THAT MAY MAKE ME DEPENDENT OR CAUSE REBOUND

This is a perception problem. Would you rather spend your afternoon feeling unwell? Migraine is a real problem, and it must be treated. If you have to take a triptan for your attacks, it's because the treatment is necessary. Make the most of modern science! As for medication-overuse headache, or rebound, it all depends on the monthly frequency of your attacks. If you have six or fewer days with attacks per month, go right ahead without hesitating; you're not at risk of medication-overuse headache. If you need a treatment on six to ten days per month, monitor yourself and consider using a preventive treatment. If you take a treatment more than ten days per month, then you are at risk of overusing and you need to limit yourself. In this case, use your eight to ten days of treatment judiciously. Treat your attacks early and try to tolerate the discomfort on subsequent days.

STATUS MIGRAINOSUS: AN ENDLESS ATTACK

In the middle of a migraine attack, the worst place to be, other than at a heavy metal concert or on a construction site, is probably a packed hospital emergency room, with its fluorescent lights, shouting people, sometimes unpleasant odours, and often very long wait time. But many migraineurs will spend time in an emergency room during their lifetime. While most migraine attacks can be brought under control by a night's sleep, some attacks last longer than seventy-two hours despite the patient's best efforts and treatments. This situation is quite common: it affects from 20 to 25 percent of migraine sufferers. For people with chronic migraine, trips to emergency can occur repeatedly.

Status migrainosus may occur in a particular context: medication withdrawal, specific stress, an active infection, etc. But sometimes no obvious trigger can be identified. The emergency room doctor's priority is then to make sure that it really is a severe migraine attack and not some other kind of headache. The doctor will use a questionnaire and physical examination to determine whether supplementary tests are needed. If the diagnosis really is migraine, then treatment is most commonly given intravenously and will usually include rehydration, a dose of an anti-inflammatory, an anti-nausea drug, and sometimes other treatments, like cortisone, narcotics, or dihydroergotamine. The success of these treatments is not guaranteed, but it's estimated that nearly 75 percent of patients leave emergency with acceptable pain relief. The headache may come back in the hours or days following, however.

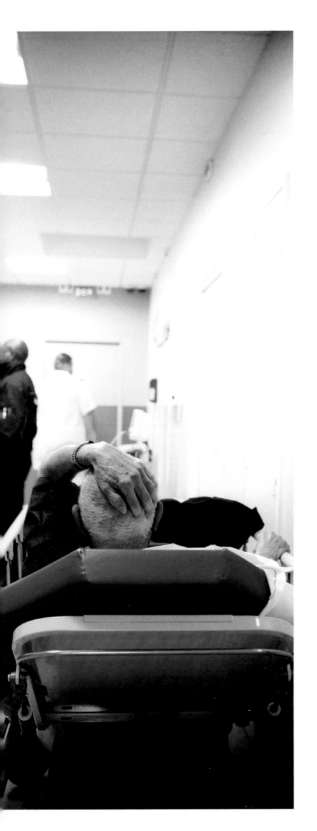

If you have gone through this extremely painful experience, it might be useful to discuss with your doctor a contingency plan, to avoid your having to go to emergency. This plan may involve specific treatments, including parenteral medications, or something other than tablets.

Attack control often remains a patient's priority. Several options are available and, with a little perseverance while trying them out, it's possible to find a satisfactory solution for treating most attacks. Over time, the warning signs become easily recognizable, and migraineurs become expert in using their treatments. While the threat of overuse is always there when attacks are frequent, it's easy to monitor by using an attack diary. In the final analysis, to kill their attacks, today's migraineurs are definitely better equipped than those of ancient Greece!

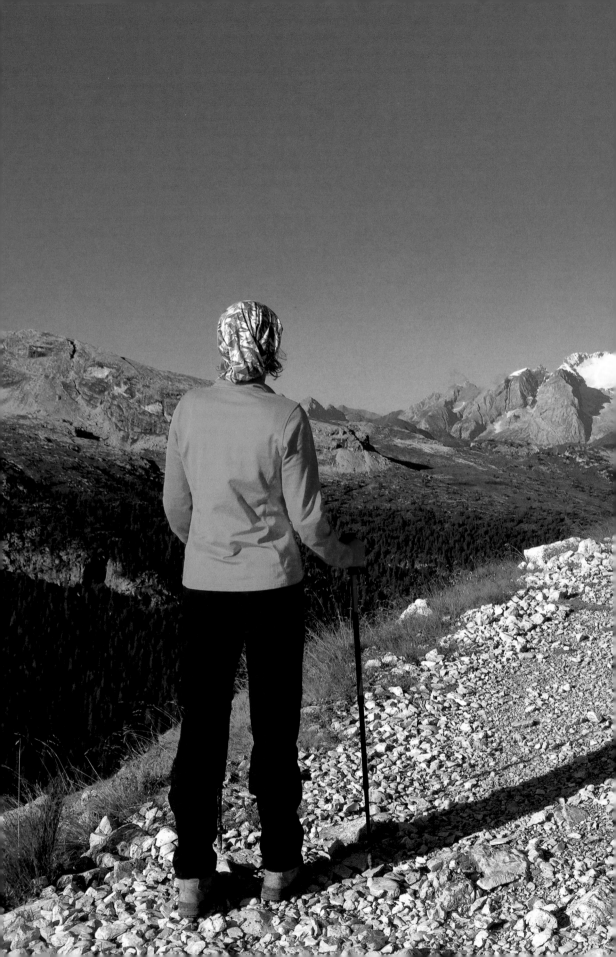

CHAPTER 8

Preventing Attacks

If you're going through hell, keep going.
— Winston Churchill

Perseverance is not a long race;
it is many short races one after the other.
— Walter Elliot

The frequency of migraine attacks varies enormously from one person to another. As we saw in Chapter 4, it may also vary throughout the lifetime of the same person. When attacks are frequent and prevent you from functioning, taking a preventive treatment may be warranted to reduce the frequency of attacks. Most people are somewhat afraid of, or even opposed to, the idea of taking these kinds of treatments. Are they dangerous? What effects do they have on the body? Will they cause dependence? Will they have side effects? Should they be taken for several years? This chapter is devoted to this important aspect of migraine management.

When Should a Preventive Treatment Be Considered?

Most patients will not deem it useful to take a preventive treatment if they have fewer than four to six days of migraine per month, especially if the attacks are well controlled. But when the number of migraine days increases to more than six to eight per month, especially if the attacks are not well controlled and they upset the normal routine for that day and perhaps the next, the situation becomes more critical. How can you function if you have to be absent from work time and again, or cancel personal activities? Of course, the decision to take a preventive treatment is the patient's — there's no absolute rule.

Can Taking a Preventive Treatment Be Avoided?

Obviously, before considering a preventive treatment, it's essential to take action on the other factors that can influence migraines. Adapting lifestyle habits is the very first step. Then, you have to ensure that the attacks are controlled as well as possible and optimize acute treatment. An attack that's properly treated from the beginning will not develop into a three-day storm. Yet even when lifestyle habits are exemplary and a suitable acute treatment has been found, the frequency of attacks may remain high and a preventive treatment will be needed.

Carole, 51

Since childhood, Carol has had migraines. For years she managed on her own. Even with two attacks a week, she was afraid to take a preventive treatment. After a series of especially painful attacks, she agreed to take amitriptyline. When she began to experience dryness in the mouth, she quite quickly stopped using it. Her doctor then recommended she try propranolol. She took it in small doses for just one month, to no effect, and decided to stop taking it too.

Discouraged, she now tells herself that nothing works. What's more, she's afraid of becoming dependent on these drugs if she takes them every day. It's better to go on putting up with the pain.... But life isn't very much fun when you're constantly threatened by an attack.

What Benefits Should Be Expected from a Preventive Treatment?

There is no treatment that entirely does away with migraines. Usually, an improvement of 50 percent in frequency and intensity is expected (Figure 54), and the remaining attacks are often easier to manage. The response rate varies from one person to another. The effect of these treatments is usually seen after they have been taken regularly for several weeks. It's therefore important to wait for two or three months before deciding on a treatment's effectiveness. Obviously, when attacks become less frequent, anxiety and

unhappiness also decrease, and it becomes easier to regain control of lifestyle habits. The ultimate goal of a preventive treatment is to improve overall quality of life.

AVAILABLE TREATMENTS

What Medications Are Most Used?

The guidelines for preventive treatment were reviewed in 2010 by the Canadian Headache Society (Figure 51). These treatments are recognized in the scientific community, since their effectiveness has been demonstrated in controlled and rigorous randomized trials. The most thoroughly tested and lowest-risk medications are used as first-line treatments. Treatments that have been the subject of fewer studies or have a less favourable side effect profile (Figure 53) are used as second- and third-line treatments. And let's not forget that sensitivity to side effects also varies from one person to another.

How Do These Treatments Work?

As we emphasized in Chapter 3, the mechanisms causing migraines are very complex and involve many brain structures and networks. It must be acknowledged that the specific action mechanisms of preventive anti-migraine treatments are poorly understood. Preventive anti-migraine treatments are all medications used to treat other medical conditions, but whose effect on migraines has sometimes been noticed by accident before being systematically studied. Among the main drug classes, antihypertensive drugs, antiepileptics, and antidepressants are used. These drugs are believed to stabilize brain activity, thus preventing the triggering of an electrical and

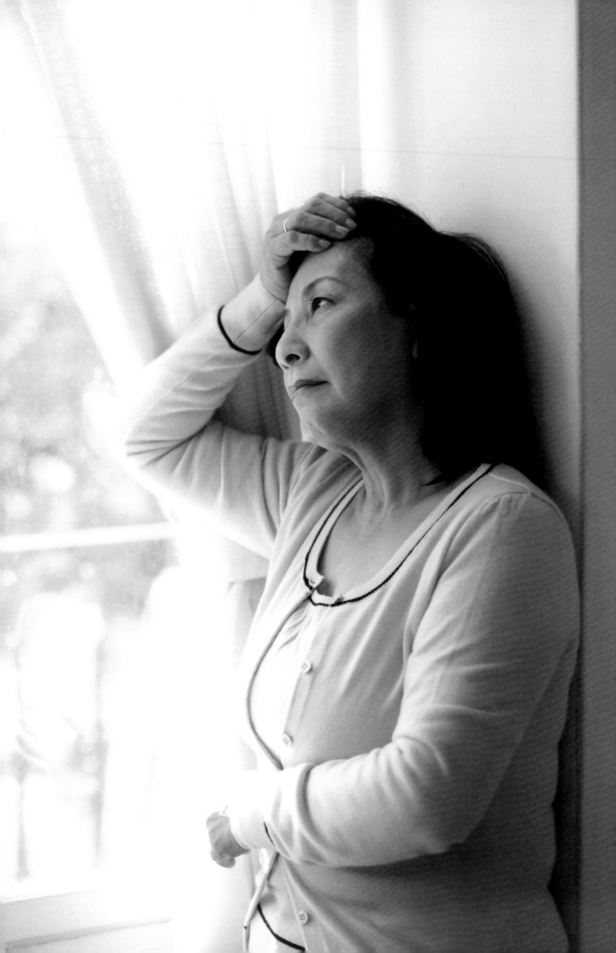

chemical migraine storm. They raise the attack trigger threshold (Figure 52). Several preventive treatments have been shown to inhibit cortical depression, the electrical brain wave that causes auras. Antidepressants enhance pain control pathways through their action on neurotransmitters like serotonin and noradrenalin.

WHAT ROLE DO NATURAL PRODUCTS PLAY?

Four natural products have been scientifically tested for migraine prevention. They are magnesium citrate, Vitamin B2 (or riboflavin), coenzyme Q10, and *Petasites hybridus*, a substance extracted from the root of the butterbur plant. The number of studies supporting these treatments is still small, and doctors tend to consider them to be low-risk options with little likelihood of side effects, but limited effectiveness. Furthermore, natural products are not medications and are therefore not covered by most insurance policies. The cost of these products may be prohibitive. Products containing combinations of different substances exist, but if they are used, it remains difficult to tell which substance is responsible for any observed positive effect. All trials of natural products should be conducted following the same rules as for standard medications.

CATEGORIES OF PREVENTIVE TREATMENTS

Category	Examples	Common Side Effects (Non-Exhaustive List)
ANTIDEPRESSANTS	Amitriptyline (Elavil) Nortriptyline (Aventyl) Venlafaxine (Effexor)	Drowsiness, dry mouth, weight gain. Nightmares, anxiety.
ANTIEPILEPTIC DRUGS	Topiramate (Topamax) Valproic Acid (Epival) Gabapentin (Neurontin)	Numbness, memory impairment, loss of appetite. Tremors, hair loss, weight gain. Drowsiness.
ANTIHYPERTENSIVE DRUGS	Propranolol (Inderal) Nadolol (Corgard) Candesartan (Atacand) Lisinopril Flunarizine (Sibelium)	Reduction of blood pressure, fainting, limited physical exercise, feeling unwell, fatigue. Dizziness, fatigue. Cough, nausea, fatigue. Depression, nightmares, weight gain.
NATURAL PRODUCTS	Magnesium Vitamin B2/riboflavin Coenzyme Q10 *Petasites hybridus*	Soft stools. Very yellow urine. Possible liver toxicity.
OTHER	Pizotifen (Sandomigran)	Drowsiness, nausea, weight gain.

FIGURE 51

Pringsheim, « Prophylactic Guidelines », *CJNS*, 2012, suppl.

IS THERE A ROLE FOR ACUPUNCTURE IN TREATING MIGRAINES?

Acupuncture has been studied for treating migraines. Treatments must be repeated regularly. High-quality studies have been carried out, and the Cochrane Group has done a systematic review summarizing the results. Acupuncture has also been compared with drug treatments. It can be concluded from this scientific literature that acupuncture treatments have a positive effect on migraines and that this effect is even comparable to that of medications. However, in studies comparing "real" acupuncture with a placebo (the insertion of needles into neutral areas, according to Chinese theories), there is no significant difference between the groups. It's therefore entirely possible that the benefits of acupuncture stem in large part from the placebo effect. It's thus up to migraine sufferers to decide if they want to try this technique, which is actually safe.

WHAT IS THE ROLE OF BOTOX IN PREVENTING MIGRAINES?

Using Botox to treat migraines may seem strange. Isn't Botox the product used by Hollywood actresses to make their wrinkles disappear? In fact, the botulinic toxin,

TRIGGER ATTACK THRESHOLD

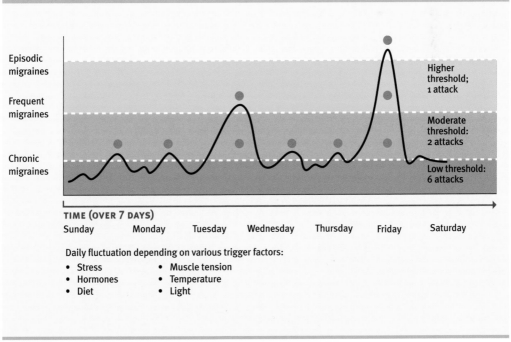

FIGURE 52

purified in a laboratory, prevents nerve endings from releasing various neurotransmitters. Its best-known effect is the muscular paralysis caused when the release of acetylcholine by motor nerves is blocked. This effect is used to treat strabismus, hyperactive bladder, spasticity, and muscle rigidity caused by damage to the nervous system. It's also used to prevent excessive sweating and hypersalivation, since botulinic toxin also inhibits gland stimulation.

The effect of Botox on headaches was noticed by chance in the 1980s, when many women in their fifties were getting Botox injections for cosmetic reasons. Some of these women — those who suffered from migraines — noted a parallel improvement in their attacks and reported this to their doctors. The first studies on Botox produced negative results, with no conclusive positive effect observed. But the patients who had participated in

them only had episodic migraine, or fewer than fifteen headache days a month. Subsequently, two major studies observed patients with chronic migraine treated with a standardized injection protocol (Figure 55). This severe type of migraine had been studied relatively little until then, as pharmaceutical companies were afraid to test medications on patients who had too many refractory headaches. However, Botox proved useful for this population, consisting of patients who had on average twenty migraine headache days a month. In 2011, Health Canada approved the use of Botox to treat chronic migraine only. As with other medications, the response rate for Botox is around 50 percent. It's neither a cure-all nor a miracle, but the benefits are sometimes impressive. There are very few side effects, which is appreciated by patients who have sometimes had various negative reactions to oral medications.

PROPHYLAXIS: TREATMENT STEPS

First line	Second line	Third line
Amitriptyline	Topiramate	Flunarizine
Propranolol	Venlafaxine	Valproate
Nadolol	Gabapentin	Botox (Chronic Migraine Only)
	Candesartan	
	Lisinopril	
	Magnesium	
	Vitamin B$_2$	
	Coenzyme Q$_{10}$	
	Butterbur	

FIGURE 53

Pringsheim, Davenport, Becker, *CMAJ*, 2010.

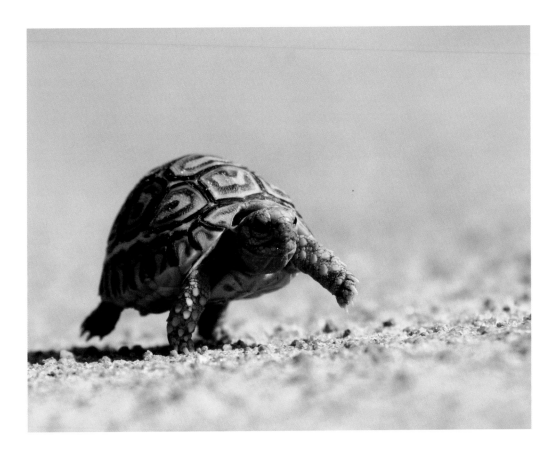

HOW SHOULD PREVENTIVE TREATMENTS BE USED?

HOW TO FIND THE RIGHT TREATMENT

It would be wonderful to be able to figure out right in the doctor's office which drug would be effective for a given patient. For the time being, however, that's impossible, and we often have to proceed by trial and error. The process of searching for an effective treatment may be long and arduous, especially when the medications tried have side effects.... It's often a veritable obstacle course. Each preventive treatment is estimated to work in 50 percent of those who try it, on average. The condition of some people will improve very noticeably, and others will derive no benefit from the treatment.

WHY KEEP A DIARY?

A diary is a must when a preventive treatment is being tried. The attacks must be clearly recorded according to how severe they are, and acute treatments taken must also be noted (see box on page 154 and Figure 32). Since the benefit of a drug is not always obvious right at the beginning, before becoming discouraged and wasting your efforts by stopping it too soon, you must be sure there are no promising signs. The dose sometimes has to be increased before the effect can be confirmed. Patience is the key to success.

WHAT ARE THE SIDE EFFECTS OF PREVENTIVE TREATMENTS?

Each treatment has different side effects (Figure 51). These usually affect fewer than 10 percent of those trying the treatment. Of course, the higher the dose, the greater the risk of side effects. In some cases, these effects can be advantageous. Let's take the case of a migraine sufferer who has trouble sleeping; the sleepiness caused by amitriptyline might be beneficial to her. Similarly, if antihypertensive drugs are given to a young woman who gets fainting spells, this will cause a problem, but if on the contrary the patient is fifty-two years old and has high blood pressure, we will kill two birds with one stone! It's the doctor's job to suggest a drug suited to your overall state of health. If side effects occur, it's sometimes wise to wait a while before you stop taking the medication. Some side effects are temporary. As is sometimes said in clinical practice, the side effects come first, the benefit comes later! If you're concerned, consult your pharmacist or doctor.

DO THESE TREATMENTS HAVE TO BE TAKEN INDEFINITELY?

If a treatment works well and improves your quality of life, your doctor will likely recommend you take it for a year. After a certain period of time, if your condition is well controlled, the treatment dose can be decreased to see if the attacks recur. If this doesn't happen, then the treatment can be stopped. But if the migraines come

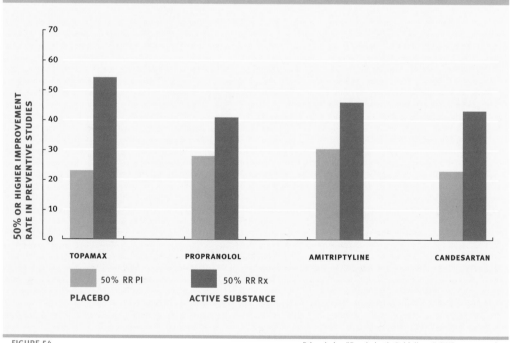

50% RESPONSE RATE IN PREVENTIVE STUDIES

FIGURE 54

Pringsheim, "Prophylactic Guidelines," *CJNS*, 2012, suppl.

back, it's definitely preferable to begin taking the treatment again. The classes of drugs suggested for migraine prevention are also used for chronic diseases like epilepsy and high blood pressure, and there is therefore a reassuring body of knowledge as to their long-term harmlessness. Many patients, especially when they're feeling better, are tempted to stop their treatment, which is entirely understandable. However, it's better to discuss this with your doctor before actually doing it, as suddenly stopping some medications may be dangerous; even more importantly, the migraines may come back worse than ever. This rebound is not always easy to control, and it's not unusual to see the situation deteriorate, even if the treatment is started again quite

quickly. There are also patients who stop their treatment because they have felt less well for several weeks. While it's possible for the treatment effect to be exhausted, it must also be remembered that migraine varies over time and that stopping a treatment during an exacerbation of attacks is likely to make the situation worse.

WILL I BECOME DEPENDENT ON THESE TREATMENTS?

Fear of dependence is very often mentioned during discussions about preventive treatments and sometimes leaves the doctor somewhat puzzled. In fact, when we compare this with other diseases, it's very rare to hear an asthmatic or a diabetic worry about developing dependence on pumps or

BOTOX INJECTION SITES FOR MIGRAINES

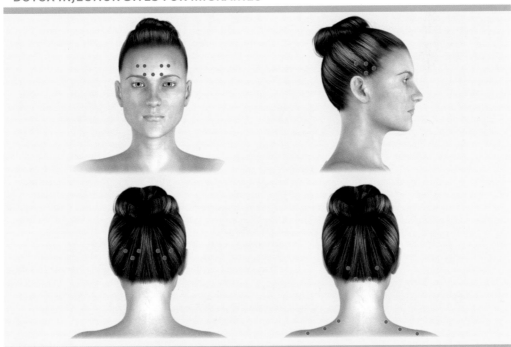

FIGURE 55

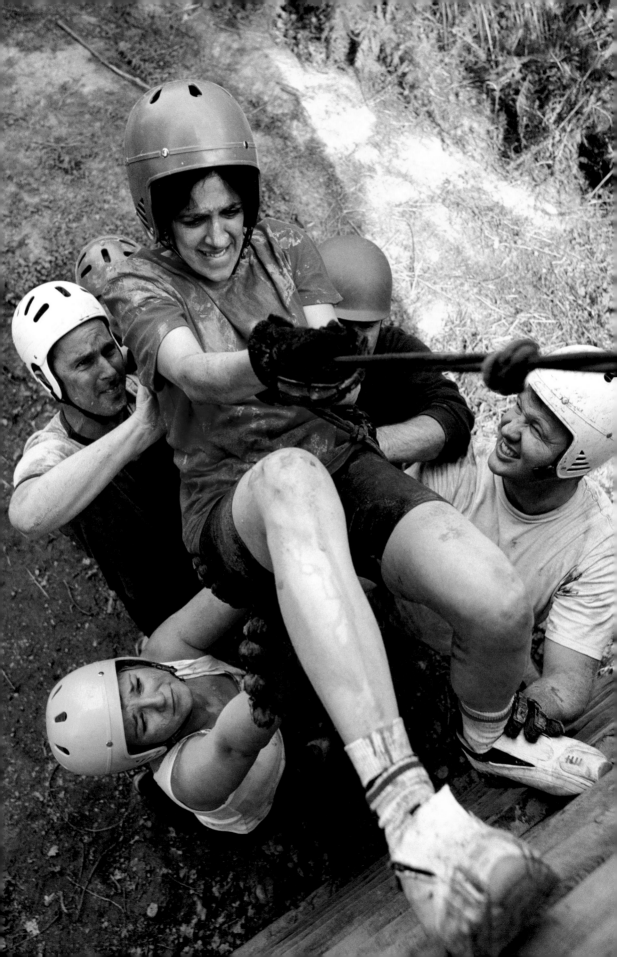

insulin. And what about people with hyperthyroidism? They will have to take replacement hormones all their lives, but does this make them dependent? It's possible that this preoccupation is related to the perception that migraine is not a "real disease." In addition, a treatment designed for the brain may raise more fears than those for other parts of the body. Is it that people are afraid their personalities will change and they'll no longer be themselves? Whatever the reason, we can say that prophylactic treatments do not cause dependence in the medical sense of the term.

WHY DOES THE TREATMENT EFFECT SOMETIMES SEEM TO WEAR OFF?

A preventive treatment may be effective in the first months of use, but after a few good months the attacks may reappear, as is often observed in clinical practice. Remember that the brain is an organ that adapts, but not always in the right direction. We know very little about the reasons underlying this "exhaustion," but it's likely that following initial stabilization other factors come into play and counteract the drug's positive effect. In this case, it's very hard to know what to do. Should the medication be stopped at the risk of seeing the situation deteriorate, or should another drug be added instead? This kind of escalation can result in a pile-up of medications that's not always beneficial.

IS COMBINING SEVERAL PREVENTIVE MEDICATIONS USEFUL?

Before considering combining treatments, they must be tried one at a time in optimal doses. This point must be emphasized, as it's common for people to become discouraged by mild side effects and abandon

Six Common Errors When Trying Preventive Treatments

1. Becoming discouraged too quickly because of side effects.

2. Not trying to increase the dosage when the drug is well tolerated.

3. Not waiting long enough before abandoning a drug. A trial should last three months.

4. Having too high expectations. The effect of most preventive treatments is a 50 percent improvement in terms of frequency.

5. Trying several preventive treatments without having gone through withdrawal in the case of medication overuse.

6. Depending entirely on medication without improving lifestyle habits and the control of other medical conditions.

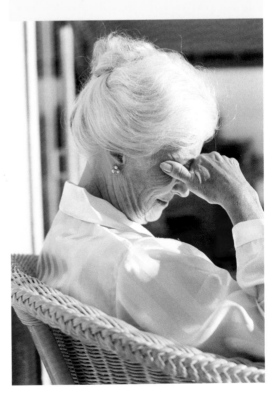

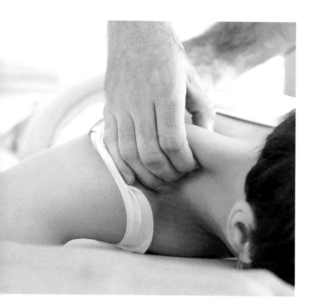

help everyone, new techniques have had to be found. Neurostimulation is based on the theory of sensory stimulation diversion. To illustrate this simple, imagine the following familiar situation: you bump your shinbone on the corner of a low table. You feel a sharp pain, and your immediate reaction is usually to rub your shin to reduce the pain. This competition between a non-painful sensation and pain occurs in both the spinal cord and the brain. This biological mechanism is sometimes called "gate control theory," as though the spinal cord, opening the gate to one sensation, had to close the gate on another. Clearly, in this example, the painful area (the shinbone) is obvious and easy to rub! A migraine attack, as described in Chapter 3, occurs in structures located inside the skull that cannot be stimulated directly. For want of a better option, many migraine sufferers tend to massage their temples, forehead, or neck during an attack. These sensations, sent to the trigeminal nucleus, compete with the painful sensations coming from the arteries and meninges.

one treatment for another. Many people thus try several treatments, but none for long enough, and then appear in the specialist's office saying they have tried everything, whereas the treatments have not been used as effectively as they could be (see box on page 157). That said, in some cases, no drug taken on its own seems to be effective enough. In such cases, the drug that's best tolerated or partially beneficial may then be combined with another. The scientific proof of the effectiveness of combinations is slim, since there have been few studies on this subject. However, owing to the large number of patients with frequent migraines, doctors recommend this approach quite often.

Many neuromodulation techniques have been used in the past and some are still in use today. Menthol pencils, for example, were already being sold in Paris at the beginning of the twentieth century, and menthol is available today in various forms — gel, creams, essential oils, etc. Our grandmothers' cold potato slices (see Chapter 7) have been replaced by complicated cooling caps. Massaging various parts of the body is recommended by acupressure specialists. Transcutaneous sensory stimulation is without doubt the most recent arrival in this family. The device is marketed in Canada under the name Cefaly.

NEUROMODULATION, A NEW APPROACH

Using electrical stimulation to fight headaches has been reported since Antiquity. In the 2000s, the neurostimulation approach has resurfaced; since medications do not

This kind of stimulation uses an electrical signal directed at the sensory nerve

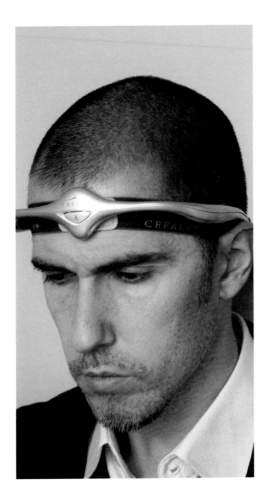

Neurostimulation can also involve electrodes implanted beneath the skin and connected to a battery that looks a lot like that of a pacemaker. The target nerves are usually the occipital nerves, but some teams also target the frontal nerves. This kind of invasive treatment was first tried in cases of cluster headache that were very hard to control. A decrease in attack frequency was observed in more than 50 percent of patients who underwent implantation. More recent studies on migraineurs have shown a modest beneficial effect on attack frequency. Currently, these techniques are only accessible in Canada in university institutes and only in very refractory cases. This surgery involves risks and requires specific expertise, as well as a close working relationship between neurologist and surgeon.

THE OBSTACLE COURSE

It's never pleasant to have to take a preventive treatment. The trial periods are often long, and not always productive. But if the attacks remain frequent, the only option is to persevere. There are many possibilities. Doctors have to supervise these attempts, but also inform and support migraine sufferers through what can only be described as an obstacle course. Most patients eventually find a solution, even though the persistence of episodic attacks often has to be accepted. For patients who still suffer, despite many tries, and who find themselves in a chronic refractory migraine situation, it's important to remain hopeful and remember that research is the only way to find new options. While waiting, the challenge is to find a balance between acceptance and being proactive!

endings in the forehead and temples. The signal is supposed to interfere with the migraine's pain signal and make the headache go away faster. A Belgian study has shown the effectiveness of this approach in preventing attacks, meaning that its regular use, even when there is no headache, leads to a decrease in the frequency of migraines. It must be stressed that patients in this study did not have very frequent migraines, on average fewer than six per month. It's thus impossible to say whether transcutaneous stimulation can improve the situation for people with more severe migraines.

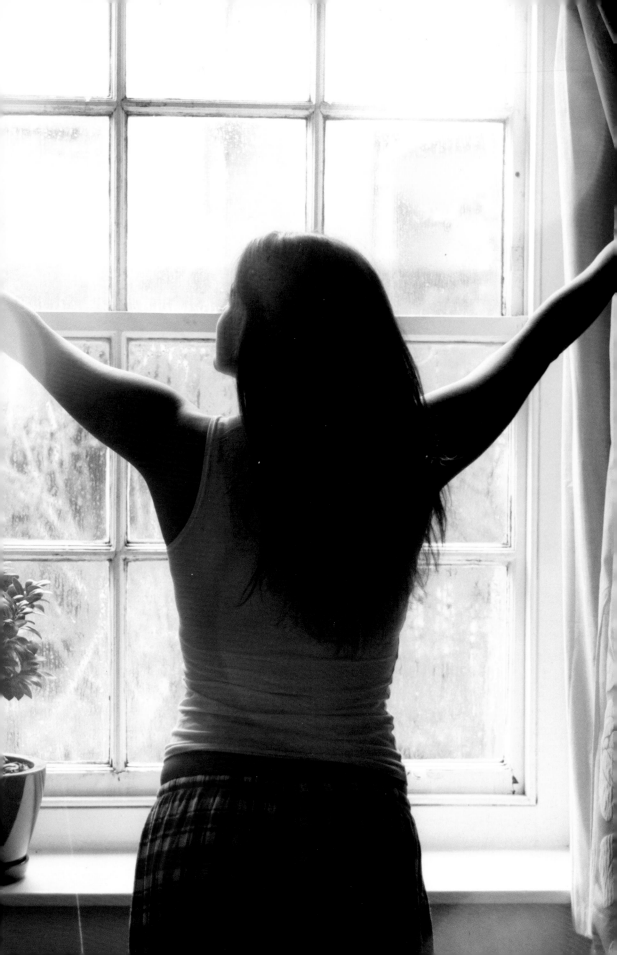

Education, Collaboration, Facilities, and Research

Migraine is a neurological disease that can take many forms, and it reflects the immense complexity of the brain. It affects so many people, in varying degrees, that it's surprising to realize that to date there are so few resources for these hundreds of thousands of people (millions worldwide). In this book, I hope I've succeeded in presenting a synthesis of historical, scientific, and epidemiological knowledge about migraine, as well as some useful basic ideas for overall management. The miracle recipe does not exist, but it must be remembered that there are a number of options.

Migraine is no longer an opaque mystery or an unavoidable curse. There have been, especially in the last fifty years, improvements, breakthroughs, and discoveries, both scientific and therapeutic. Associations have been established. Websites have been created. Patients are telling their stories. Research is underway. We've come a long way, but we have a long way to go.

Yet, as I described in the Introduction, there are still too many people who suffer in silence, sometimes for years, despite the existence of treatments. The problem of access to care is fundamental and especially affects migraineurs. As a result, we have to do better … and it's encouraging to realize we can do better.

The Canadian Migraine Strategy, published in 2010, painted a realistic picture of the situation with respect to migraine in Canada and proposed detailed solutions — the creation of centres of excellence in the field of headaches, for example. Of course, these centres will never be able to see everyone with migraines, but they should become hubs for influencing the entire health network, through training as well as in other ways.

Education is at the heart of this strategy. Doctors must be better trained, as must other professionals who may be able to help migraine sufferers: nurses, pharmacists, physiotherapists, occupational therapists, psychologists, etc. If migraineurs are to play a role in their own care, they must have access to reliable general information, as well as to more detailed resources adapted to their specific situation. Employers have to better understand the impact of migraines on their employees' functioning. Politicians and decision-makers must be sensitized to the importance of this disease and allocate funds for care and care facilities. The social stigma connected with migraine must be eliminated. Myths, perpetuated for hundreds of years, must be dismantled, one by one. Understanding and education must replace discouragement and passivity. Available treatments must become accessible.

And let's not forget research. Even in the best clinics, with the help of the most expert specialists, current treatments do not succeed in helping all migraineurs. People with chronic refractory migraine know what I'm talking about. The development of research teams, both fundamental and clinical, must be part of the plan. Examples of the critical importance of research are not lacking, whether in the field of coronary disease, cancer, state-of-the-art surgery ... it's by increasing our knowledge that new treatments are developed.

So we have our work cut out for us! There are facilities to establish, groups to set up, and collaborative efforts to get underway. In a hospital or in a clinic, this is a team effort. On a larger scale, this is a task for society and for political decision-makers. But everything invariably begins with people and their families. If migraine is getting you down, or if you know someone close to you who suffers from it, it isn't enough to get discouraged or be offended by waiting lists. Get informed, get involved, ask your questions, share your knowledge. Look for support. Give support. Be positive. In difficult moments, tell yourself over and over again that giving up is not an option.

But, above all, remember one thing: if you have migraines, you're not alone!

Elizabeth Leroux, M.D., FRCPC

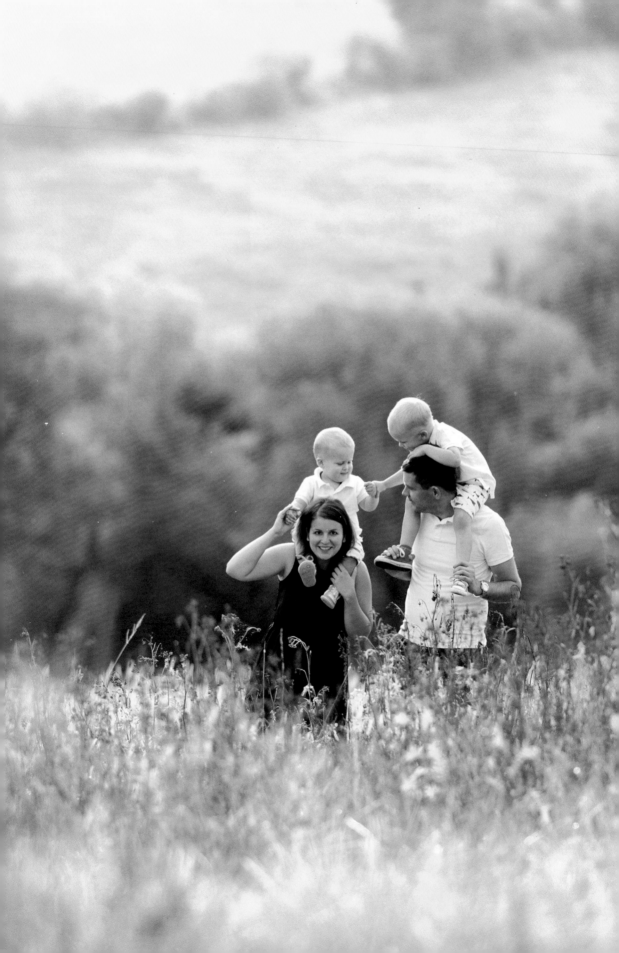

About the Author

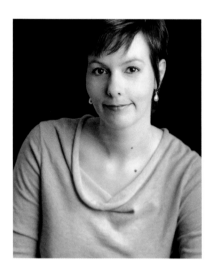

Born in Montreal in 1978, Elizabeth Leroux graduated in medicine from the Université de Montreal. During her neurology residency, she began to be interested in headaches. Dr. Leroux spent a year practising in Rouyn-Noranda, before specializing in headache medicine in Paris, at Le Centre d'Urgence Céphalées at Hôpital Lariboisière. She then published research studies on cluster headache. Returning to Montreal in 2010, she joined the migraine clinic at Centre Hospitalier de l'Université de Montréal, where she is now director. Involved in the management of complex cases, as well as in teaching and research, she is working on expanding the clinic.

An active member of the Canadian Headache Society, Dr. Leroux is responsible for the Canadian headache course for residents in neurology. She regularly lectures on headaches, both to the general public and to healthcare professionals. Convinced that it's possible to provide more help to people with migraines and other types of headaches, she has created the Migraine Québec website, now a non-profit, charitable organization (www.migrainequebec.com).

To Learn More ...

Chapter 1

Amoozegar, F., D. Guglielmin, W. Hu, D. Chan, and W.J. Becker. "Spontaneous Intracranial Hypotension: Recommendations for Management." *The Canadian Journal of Neurological Sciences* 40, no. 2 (2013): 144–57.

Boisselle, C., R. Guthmann, and K. Cable. "Clinical Inquiry. What Clinical Clues Differentiate Migraine from Sinus Headaches? Pulsatile Quality, Duration of 4 to 72 Hours, Unilateral Location, Nausea or Vomiting, and Disabling Intensity." *The Journal of Family Practice* 62, no. 12 (2013): 752–54.

Crystal, S.C., and M.S. Robbins. "Epidemiology of Tension-Type Headache." *Current Pain and Headache Reports* 14, no. 6 (2010): 449–54.

Dodick, D. "Diagnosing Headache: Clinical Clues and Clinical Rules." *Advanced Studies in Medicine* 3, no. 2 (2003): 87–92.

Elliot, S., and D. Kernick. "Why Do GPs with a Special Interest in Headache Investigate Headache Presentations with Neuroradiology and What Do They Find?" *The Journal of Headache Pain* 12, no. 6 (2011): 625–28.

Eross, E., D. Dodick, and M. Eross. "The Sinus, Allergy and Migraine Study (SAMS)." *Headache* 47, no. 2 (2007): 213–24.

Friedman, D.I. "The Pseudotumor Cerebri Syndrome." *Neuralgic Clinics* 32, no. 2 (2014): 363–96.

Gantenbein, A.R., C. Jaggi et al. "Awareness of Headache and of National Headache Society Activities among Primary Care Physicians — A Qualitative Study." *BMC Research Notes* 6 (2013): 118.

Gladstone, J. "From Psychoneurosis to ICHD-2: An Overview of the State of the Art in Post-Traumatic Headache." *Headache* 49, no. 7 (2009): 1097–111.

Hamilton, W., and D. Kernick. "Clinical Features of Primary Brain Tumours: A Case-Control Study Using Electronic Primary Care Records." *The British Journal of General Practice* 57, no. 542 (2007): 695–99.

Herrero-Velazquez, S., M.I. Pedraza et al. "Referrals from Primary Care to a Dedicated Headache Clinic: Analysis of the First 1,000 Patients." *La Revue neurologique* 58, no. 11 (2014): 487–92.

Howard, L., S. Wessely et al. "Are Investigations Anxiolytic or Anxiogenic? A Randomised Controlled Trial of Neuroimaging to Provide Reassurance in Chronic Daily Headache." *The Journal of Neurology, Neurosurgery, and Psychiatry* 76, no. 11 (2005): 1558–564.

The International Classification of Headache Disorders. 3rd edition (beta version). *Cephalalgia* 33, no. 9 (2013): 629–808.

Kaniecki, R.G. "Tension-Type Headache." *Continuum* 18, no. 4 (2012): 823–34.

KERNICK, D.P., F. AHMED et al. "Imaging Patients with Suspected Brain Tumour: Guidance for Primary Care." *The British Journal of General Practice* 58, no. 557 (2008): 880–85.

LIPTON, R.B., D. DODICK et al. "A self-administered screener for migraine in primary care: The ID Migraine validation study." Neurology 61, no. 3 (2003): 375-82.

LIPTON, R.B., W.F. STEWART, D.D. CELENTANO, and M.L. REED. "Undiagnosed Migraine Headaches. A Comparison of Symptom-Based and Reported Physician Diagnosis." *Archives of Internal Medicine* 152, no. 6 (1992): 1273–78.

MORRIS, Z., W.N. WHITELEY et al. "Incidental Findings on Brain Magnetic Resonance Imaging: Systematic Review and Meta-Analysis." *BMJ* 339 (2009): b3016.

PEDERSEN, J.L., M. BARLOESE, and R.H. JENSEN. "Neurostimulation in Cluster Headache: A Review of Current Progress." *Cephalalgia* 33, no. 14 (2013): 1179–93.

PRAKASH, S. "New Daily Persistent Headache: Disease or Syndrome?" *Headache* 53, no. 4 (2013): 678–79.

ROBBINS, M.S., D. KURUVILLA et al. "Trigger Point Injections for Headache Disorders: Expert Consensus Methodology and Narrative Review." *Headache* 54, no. 9 (2014): 1441–59.

ROBBINS, M.S., and R.W. EVANS. "The Heterogeneity of New Daily Persistent Headache." *Headache* 52, no. 10 (2012): 1579–89.

SANDRINI, G., L. FRIBERG et al. "Neurophysiological Tests and Neuroimaging Procedures in Non-Acute Headache (2nd edition)." *European Journal of Neurology* 18, no. 3 (2011): 373–81.

WEAVER-AGOSTONI, J. "Cluster Headache." *American Family Physician* 88, no. 2 (2013): 122–28.

YUH, E.L., G.W. HAWRYLUK, and G.T. MANLEY. "Imaging Concussion: A Review." *Neurosurgery* 75, Supplement 4 (2014): S50–63.

ZAKRZEWSKA, J.M., and M.E. LINSKEY. "Trigeminal Neuralgia." *BMJ* 348 (2014): g474.

Chapter 2

BECKER, W.J., S.N. CHRISTIE, G. MACKIE, and P. COOPER. "Consensus Statement: The Development of a National Canadian Migraine Strategy." *Canadian Journal of Neuroscience* 37, no. 4 (2010): 449–56.

BIGAL, M.E. AND M.A. ARRUDA. "Migraine in the Pediatric Population — Evolving Concepts." *Headache* 50, no. 7 (2010): 1130–43.

BORHANI HAGHIGHI, A., S. MOTAZEDIAN, and R. REZAII. "Therapeutic Potentials of Menthol in Migraine Headache: Possible Mechanisms of Action." *Medical Hypotheses* 69, no. 2 (2007): 455.

BUSE, D. "13 Things Not to Say to Someone with a Migraine." *Huffington Post*, October 2, 2014.

COLLADO-VAZQUEZ, S. and J.M. CARRILLO. "Cranial Trepanation in the Egyptian." *Neurologia* 29, no. 7 (2014): 433–40.

COOKE, L.J. and W.J. BECKER. "Migraine Prevalence, Treatment and Impact: The Canadian Women and Migraine Study." *Canadian Journal of Neuroscience* 37, no. 5 (2010): 580–87.

DEER, T. R., N. MEKHAIL et al. "The Appropriate Use of Neurostimulation: Stimulation of the Intracranial and Extracranial Space and Head for Chronic Pain." *Neuromodulation* 17, no. 6 (2014): 551–70; discussion 570.

EVANS, R.W., R.B. LIPTON, and S.D. SILBERSTEIN. "The Prevalence of Migraine in Neurologists." *Neurology* 61, no. 9 (2003): 1271–72.

FURMANSKI, A.R. "Dynamic Concepts of Migraine; A Character Study of One Hundred Patients." *AMA Archives of Neurology and Psychiatry* 67, no. 1 (1952): 23–31.

GUSTAVSSON, A., M. SVENSSON et al. "Cost of Disorders of the Brain in Europe 2010." *European Neuro-psychopharmacology* 21, no. 10 (2011): 718–79.

KOEHLER, P.J. and C.J. BOES. "A History of Non-Drug Treatment in Headache, Particularly Migraine." *Brain* 133 (Pt 8) (2010): 2489–500.

LOFLAND, J.H., and K.D. FRICK. "Workplace Absenteeism and Aspects of Access to Health Care for Individuals with Migraine Headache." *Headache* 46, no. 4 (2006): 563–76.

MAGIORKINIS, E., A. DIAMANTIS, D.D. MITSIKOSTAS, and G. ANDROUTSOS. "Headaches in Antiquity and During the Early Scientific Era." *Journal of Neurology* 256, no. 8 (2009): 1215–20.

MANSOUR, K.J. "Migraine: Dynamics and Choice of Symptom." *Psychoanalysis Q* 26, no. 4 (1957): 476–93.

MERIKANGAS, K.R. "Contributions of Epidemiology to Our Understanding of Migraine." *Headache* 53, no. 2 (2013): 230–46.

RAMAGE-MORIN, P.L., and H. GILMOUR. "Prevalence of Migraine in the Canadian Household Population." *Health Report* 25, no. 6 (2014): 10–16.

SACKS, O. "Migraine." *Édition revue et augmentée.* Paris: Éditions du Seuil, 1996.

VOS, T., A.D. FLAXMAN et al. "Years Lived with Disability (YLDS) for 1160 Sequelae of 289 Diseases and Injuries 1990–2010: A Systematic Analysis for the Global Burden of Disease Study 2010." *Lancet* 380, no. 9859 (2012): 2163–96.

YOUNG, W.B., J.E. PARK, I.X. TIAN, and J. KEMPNER. "The Stigma of Migraine." *PLoS One* 8, no. 1 (2013): e54074.

Chapter 3

AHN, A.H., and K.C. BRENNAN. "Unanswered Questions in Headache: How Does a Migraine Attack Stop?" *Headache* 52, no. 1 (2012): 186–87.

BOGDUK, N., and J. GOVIND. "Cervicogenic Headache: An Assessment of the Evidence on Clinical Diagnosis, Invasive Tests, and Treatment." *Lancet* 8, no. 10 (2009): 959–68.

CHAI, N.C., R.E. SHAPIRO, and A.M. RAPOPORT. "Why Does Vomiting Stop a Migraine Attack?" *Current Pain Headache Report* 17, no. 9 (2013): 362.

CHARLES, A.C., and S.M. BACA. "Cortical Spreading Depression and Migraine." *Nature Reviews Neurology* 9, no. 11 (2013): 637-44.

DALKARA, T., A. NOZARI, and M.A. MOSKOWITZ. "Migraine Aura Pathophysiology: The Role of Blood Vessels and Microembolisation." *Lancet Neurology* 9, no. 3 (2010): 309–17.

DIGRE, K.B., and K.C. BRENNAN "Shedding Light on Photophobia." *Journal of Neuro-Ophthalmology* 32, no. 1 (2012): 68–81.

GEPPETTI, P., E. ROSSI, A. CHIARUGI, and S. BENEMEI. "Antidromic Vasodilatation and the Migraine Mechanism." *Journal of Headache Pain* 13, no. 2 (2012): 103–11.

GOADSBY, P.J., R.B. LIPTON, and M.D. FERRARI. "Migraine — Current Understanding and Treatment." *The New England Journal of Medicine* 346, no. 4 (2002): 257–70.

HARRIOTT, A.M., and T.J. SCHWEDT. "Migraine Is Associated with Altered Processing of Sensory Stimuli." *Current Pain Headache Report* 18, no. 11 (2014): 458.

KELMAN, L. "The Aura: A Tertiary Care Study of 952 Migraine Patients." *Cephalalgia* 24, no. 9 (2004): 728–34.

KELMAN, L. "The Premonitory Symptoms (Prodrome): A Tertiary Care Study of 893 Migraineurs." *Headache* 44, no. 9 (2004): 865–72.

LIPTON, R.B., M.E. BIGAL et al. "Cutaneous Allodynia in the Migraine Population." *Annals of Neurology* 63, no. 2 (2008): 148–58.

LODER, E. "What is the Evolutionary Advantage of Migraine?" *Cephalalgia* 22, no. 8 (2002): 624–32.

MAGIS, D., A. VIGANO et al. "Pearls and Pitfalls: Electrophysiology for Primary Headaches." *Cephalalgia* 33, no. 8 (2013): 526–39.

MANIYAR, F.H., T. SPRENGER, T. MONTEITH, C. SCHANKIN, and P.J. GOADSBY. "Brain Activations in the Premonitory Phase of Nitroglycerin-Triggered Migraine Attacks." *Brain* 137 (Pt 1) (2014): 232–41.

MAY, A. "Pearls and Pitfalls: Neuroimaging in Headache." *Cephalalgia* 33, no. 8 (2013): 554–65.

NOSEDA, R., and R. BURSTEIN "Migraine Pathophysiology: Anatomy of the Trigeminovascular Pathway and Associated Neurological Symptoms, Cortical Spreading Depression, Sensitization, and Modulation of Pain." *Pain* 154, Supplement 1 (2013): S44–53.

PEROUTKA, S.J. "Neurogenic Inflammation and Migraine: Implications for the Therapeutics." *Molecular Intervention* 5, no. 5 (2005): 304–11.

QUEIROZ, L.P., D.I. FRIEDMAN, A.M. RAPOPORT, and R.A. PURDY. "Characteristics of Migraine Visual Aura in Southern Brazil and Northern USA." *Cephalalgia* 31, no. 16 (2011): 1652–58.

SILBERSTEIN, S.D. and D.W. DODICK. "Migraine Genetics: Part II." *Headache* 53, no. 8 (2013): 1218–29.

SILVA-NETO, R.P., M.F. PERES, and M.M. VALENCA. "Accuracy of Osmophobia in the Differential Diagnosis Between Migraine And Tension-Type Headache." *Journal of Neurological Science* 339, nos. 1–2 (2014): 118–22.

STOLTE, B., D. HOLLE, S. NAEGEL, H.C. DIENER, and M. OBERMANN. "Vestibular Migraine." *Cephalalgia* 35, no. 3 (2014): 262–70.

TFELT-HANSEN, P.C., and P.J. KOEHLER. "One Hundred Years of Migraine Research: Major Clinical and Scientific Observations from 1910 to 2010." *Headache* 51, no. 5 (2011): 752–78.

Chapter 4

ADAMS, A.M., D. SERRANO et al. "The Impact of Chronic Migraine: The Chronic Migraine Epidemiology and Outcomes (CaMEO) Study Methods and Baseline Results." *Cephalalgia* 35, no. 7 (2014): 563–78.

BIGAL, M.E., and R.B. LIPTON. "What Predicts the Change from Episodic to Chronic Migraine?" *Current Opinion in Neurology* 22, no. 3 (2009): 269–76.

DIENER, H.C., D.W. DODICK et al. "Chronic Migraine — Classification, Characteristics and Treatment." *Nature Reviews Neurology* 8, no. 3 (2011): 162–71.

KRISTOFFERSEN, E.S., and C. LUNDQVIST. "Medication-Overuse Headache: A Review." *Journal of Pain Research* 7 (2014): 367–78.

LODER, E., E. WEIZENBAUM, B. FRISHBERG, and S. SILBERSTEIN. "Choosing Wisely in Headache Medicine: The American Headache Society's List of Five Things Physicians and Patients Should Question." *Headache* 53, no. 10 (2013): 1651–59.

MACGREGOR, E.A. "Prevention and Treatment of Menstrual Migraine." *Drugs* 70, no. 14 (2010): 1799–818.

MANACK, A., D.C. BUSE, D. SERRANO, C.C. TURKEL, and R.B. LIPTON. "Rates, Predictors, and Consequences of Remission from Chronic Migraine to Episodic Migraine." *Neurology* 76, no. 8 (2011): 711–18.

NOSEDA, R., V. KAINZ, D. BORSOOK, and R. BURSTEIN. "Neurochemical Pathways That Converge on Thalamic Trigeminovascular Neurons: Potential Substrate for Modulation of Migraine by Sleep, Food Intake, Stress and Anxiety." *PLoS One* 9, no. 8 (2014): e103929.

PRINGSHEIM, T., W.J. DAVENPORT, and D. DODICK. "Acute Treatment and Prevention of Menstrually Related Migraine Headache: Evidence-Based Review." *Neurology* 70, no. 17 (2008): 1555–63.

SCHULMAN, E. "Refractory Migraine — A Review." *Headache* 53, no. 4 (2013): 599–613.

TEPPER, S.J., and D.E. TEPPER. "Breaking the Cycle of Medication Overuse Headache." *Cleveland Clinic Journal of Medicine* 77, no. 4 (2010): 236–42.

TIETJEN, G.E., and B.L. Peterlin. "Childhood Abuse and Migraine: Epidemiology, Sex Differences, and Potential Mechanisms." *Headache* 51, no. 6 (2011): 869–79.

TIETJEN, G.E., N.A. HERIAL, J. HARDGROVE, C. UTLEY, and L. WHITE. "Migraine Comorbidity Constellations." *Headache* 47, no. 6 (2007): 857–65.

Chapter 5

BENEDETTI, F. "Placebo and the New Physiology of the Doctor-Patient Relationship." *Physiological Review* 93, no. 3 (2013): 1207–46.

BUSE, D.C., M.F. RUPNOW, and R.B. LIPTON. "Assessing and Managing All Aspects of Migraine: Migraine Attacks, Migraine-Related Functional Impairment, Common Comorbidities, and Quality of Life." *Mayo Clinic Proceedings* 84, no. 5 (2009): 422–35.

CHAI, N.C., B.L. PETERLIN, and A.H. CALHOUN. "Migraine and Estrogen." *Current Opinion in Neurology* 27, no. 3 (2014): 315–24.

DAVANZO, R., J. BUA, G. PALONI, and G. FACCHINA. "Breastfeeding and Migraine Drugs." *European Journal of Clinical Pharmacology* 70, no. 11 (2014): 1313–24.

DODICK, D. "Patient Perceptions and Treatment Preferences in Migraine Management." *CNS Drugs* 16, Supplement 1 (2002): 19–24.

EDMEADS, J. "Communication Issues in Migraine Diagnosis." *Canadian Journal of Neurological Sciences* 29, Supplement 2 (2002): S8–10.

HALL, K.T., and T.J. KAPTCHUK. "Genetic biomarkers of Placebo Response: What Could it Mean for Future Trial Design?" *Clinical Investigations* (London) 3, no. 4 (2013): 311–14.

HORING, B., K. WEIMER, E.R., MUTH, and P. ENCK. "Prediction of Placebo Responses: A Systematic Review of the Literature." *Frontiers in Psychology* 5 (2014): 1079.

IBRAHIMI, K., E.G. COUTURIER, and A. MAASSEN-VANDENBRINK. "Migraine and Perimenopause." *Maturitas* 78, no. 4 (2014): 277–80.

KINDELAN-CALVO, P., A. GIL-MARTINEZ et al. "Effectiveness of Therapeutic Patient Education for Adults with Migraine. A Systematic Review and Meta-Analysis of Randomized Controlled Trials." *Pain Medicine* 15, no. 9 (2014): 1619–36.

MACGREGOR, E.A. "Migraine in Pregnancy and Lactation." *Neurological Sciences* 35, Supplement 1 (2014): 61–64.

MEISSNER, K., M. FASSLER et al. "Differential Effectiveness of Placebo Treatments: A Systematic Review of Migraine Prophylaxis." *JAMA International Medicine* 173, no. 21 (2013): 1941–51.

PURDY, R.A. "Migraine: The Doctor-Patient Link. Results of a Needs Assessment." *Canadian Journal of Neurological Sciences* 29, Supplement 2 (2002): S3–7.

SHEFTELL, F.D. "Communicating the Right Therapy for the Right Patient at the Right Time: Acute Therapy." *Canadian Journal of Neurological Sciences* 29, Supplement 2 (2002): S33–39.

Chapter 6

ANDRASIK, F. "Biofeedback in Headache: An Overview of Approaches and Evidence." *Cleveland Clinic Journal of Medicine* 77, Supplement 3 (2010): S72–76.

"Aux origines de la méditation." *Le Point*, numéro hors série, juillet-août 2014.

BALDACCI, F., M. VEDOVELLO et al. "How Aware Are Migraineurs of their Triggers?" *Headache* 53, no. 5 (2013): 834–37.

BIGAL, M.E., and A.M. RAPOPORT. "Obesity and Chronic Daily Headache." *Current Pain and Headache Reports* 16, no. 1 (2012): 101–09.

BIGAL, M.E., J.N. LIBERMAN, and R.B. LIPTON. "Obesity and Migraine: A Population Study." *Neurology* 66, no. 4 (2006): 545–50.

BLAU, J.N. "Water Deprivation: A New Migraine Precipitant." *Headache* 45, no. 6 (2005): 757–59.

CADY, R.K., K. FARMER, J.K. DEXTER, and J. HALL. "The Bowel and Migraine: Update on Celiac Disease and Irritable Bowel Syndrome." *Current Pain and Headache Reports* 16, no. 3 (2012): 278–86.

CALHOUN, A.H., and S. FORD. "Behavioral Sleep Modification May Revert Transformed Migraine to Episodic Migraine." *Headache* 47, no. 8 (2007): 1178–83.

COLLURA, T.F., and R.W. THATCHER. "Clinical Benefit to Patients Suffering from Recurrent Migraine Headaches and Who Opted to Stop Medication and Take a Neurofeedback Treatment Series." *Clinical EEG and Neuroscience* 42, no. 2 (2011): VIII–IX.

DE LUCA CANTO, G., V. SINGH, M.E. BIGAL, P.W. MAJOR, and C. FLORES-MIR. "Association Between Tension-Type Headache and Migraine with Sleep Bruxism: A Systematic Review." *Headache* 54, no. 9 (2014): 1460–69.

DE TOMMASO, M., M. DELUSSI et al. "Sleep Features and Central Sensitization Symptoms in Primary Headache Patients." *Journal of Headache and Pain* 15 (2014): 64.

DIMITROVA, A.K., R.C. UNGARO et al. "Prevalence of Migraine in Patients with Celiac Disease and Inflammatory Bowel Disease." *Headache* 53, no. 2 (2013): 344–55.

FREEDOM, T., AND R.W. EVANS. "Headache and Sleep." *Headache* 53, no. 8 (2013): 1358–66.

GOLDSTEIN, J., M. HAGEN, and M. GOLD. "Results of a Multicenter, Double-Blind, Randomized, Parallel-Group, Placebo-Controlled, Single-Dose Study Comparing the Fixed Combination of Acetaminophen, Acetylsalicylic Acid, and Caffeine with Ibuprofen for Acute Treatment of Patients with Severe Migraine." *Cephalalgia* 34, no. 13 (2014): 1070–78.

Gori, S., C. Lucchesi et al. "Sleep-Related Migraine Occurrence Increases with Aging." *Acta Neurol Belg* 112, no. 2 (2012): 183–87.

HABA-RUBIO, J., M. TAFTI, R. HEINZER, D.S. BOND, and R.R. WING. "Improvement of Migraine Headaches in Severely Obese Patients After Bariatric Surgery." *Neurology* 77, no. 19 (2011): 1772–73; author reply 1773.

HOY, S.M., and L.J. SCOTT. "Indomethacin/Prochlorperazine/Caffeine: A Review of Its Use in the Acute Treatment of Migraine and in the Treatment of Episodic Tension-Type Headache." *CNS Drugs* 25, no. 4 (2011): 343–58.

INALOO, S., S.M. DEHGHANI, F. FARZADI, M. HAGHIGHAT, and M.H. IMANIEH. "A Comparative Study of Celiac Disease in Children with Migraine Headache and a Normal Control Group." *Turkish Journal of Gastroenterology* 22, no. 1 (2011): 32–35.

JOHN, P.J., N. SHARMA, C.M. SHARMA, and A. KANKANE. "Effectiveness of Yoga Therapy in the Treatment of Migraine Without Aura: A Randomized Controlled Trial." *Headache* 47, no. 5 (2014): 654–61.

KANKANE, A. "Efficacy of Yoga in Treatment of Migraine." *Annals of Indian Academy of Neurology* 16, no. 3 (2013): 462–63.

KISAN, R., M. Sujan et al. "Effect of Yoga on Migraine: A Comprehensive Study Using Clinical Profile and Cardiac Autonomic Functions." *International Journal of Yoga* 7, no. 2 (2014): 126–32.

KOSEOGLU, E., M.F. YETKIN, F. UGUR, AND M. BILGEN. "The Role of Exercise in Migraine Treatment Short Title: Exercise in Migraine." *Journal of Sports Medicine and Physical Fitness* (2014).

LIPTON, R.B., D.C. BUSE et al. "Reduction in Perceived Stress as a Migraine Trigger: Testing the 'Let-Down Headache' Hypothesis." *Neurology* 82, no. 16 (2014): 1395–401.

LUCCHESI, L.M., J.G. SPECIALI et al. "Nocturnal Awakening with Headache and Its Relationship with Sleep Disorders in a Population-Based Sample of Adult Inhabitants of Sao Paulo City, Brazil." *Cephalalgia* 30, no. 12 (2010): 1477–85.

MARCUS, D.A., L. SCHARFF, D. TURK, and L.M. GOURLEY. "A Double-Blind Provocative Study of Chocolate as a Trigger of Headache." *Cephalalgia* 17, no. 8 (1997): 855–62; discussion 800.

MARTINS, I.P., and R.G. GOUVEIA. "More on Water and Migraine." *Cephalalgia* 27, no. 4 (2007): 372–74.

MYERS, K.A., M. MRKOBRADA, and D.L. SIMEL. "Does This Patient Have Obstructive Sleep Apnea?: The Rational Clinical Examination Systematic Review." *JAMA* 310, no. 7 (2013): 731–41.

NASSINI, R., S. MATERAZZI et al. "The 'Headache Tree' Via Umbellulone and TRPA1 Activates the Trigeminovascular System." *Brain* 135 (Pt 2) (2012): 376–90.

NESBITT, A.D., G.D. LESCHZINER, and R.C. PEATFIELD. "Headache, Drugs and Sleep." *Cephalalgia* 34, no. 10 (2014): 756–66.

PEROUTKA, S.J. "What Turns On a Migraine? A Systematic Review of Migraine Precipitating Factors." *Current Pain and Headache Reports* 18, no. 10 (2014): 454.

PFALLER, A. "Efficacy of Biofeedback in the Treatment of Migraine and Tension Type Headaches." *Pain Physician* 13, no. 1 (2010): 94–96; author reply 96.

RAINS, J.C., and J.S. POCETA. "Sleep and Headache Disorders: Clinical Recommendations for Headache Management." *Headache* 46, Supplement 3 (2006): S147–148.

ROCKETT, F.C., V.R. DE OLIVEIRA et al. "Dietary Aspects of Migraine Trigger Factors." *Nutrition Reviews* 70, no. 6 (2012): 337–56.

RUSSELL, M.B., H.A. KRISTIANSEN, and K.J. KVAERNER. "Headache in Sleep Apnea Syndrome: Epidemiology and Pathophysiology." *Cephalalgia* 34, no. 10 (2014): 752–55.

SARACCO, M.G., G. CALABRESE et al. "Relationship Between Primary Headache and Nutrition: A Questionnaire about Dietary Habits of Patients with Headache." *Neurological Sciences* 35, Supplement 1 (2014): 159–61.

SPIERINGS, E.L., S. DONOGHUE, A. MIAN, and C. WOBER. "Sufficiency and Necessity in Migraine: How Do We Figure Out if Triggers Are Absolute or Partial and, if Partial, Additive or Potentiating." *Current Pain and Headache Reports* 18, no. 10 (2014): 455.

STOKES, D.A., and M.S. LAPPIN. "Neurofeedback and Biofeedback with 37 Migraineurs: A Clinical Outcome Study." *Behavioural and Brain Functions* 6 (2010): 9.

TAVARES, C., and R.K. SAKATA. "Caffeine in the Treatment of Pain." *Revista Brasileira de Anestesiologia* 62, no. 3 (2012): 387–401.

WELLS, R.E., R. BURCH et al. "Meditation for Migraines: A Pilot Randomized Controlled Trial." *Headache* 54, no. 9 (2014): 1484–95.

Chapter 7

BARON, E.P., S.Y. MARKOWITZ et al. "Triptan Education and Improving Knowledge for Optimal Migraine Treatment: An Observational Study." *Headache* 54, no. 4 (2014): 686–97.

DAHLOF, C.G. "Infrequent or Non-Response to Oral Sumatriptan Does Not Predict Response to Other Triptans — Review of Four Trials." *Cephalalgia* 26, no. 2 (2006): 98–106.

DIAZ-INSA, S.P., J. GOADSBY et al. "The Impact of Allodynia on the Efficacy of Almotriptan when Given Early in Migraine: Data from the 'Act When Mild' Study." *International Journal of Neuroscience* 121, no. 12 (2011): 655–61.

DODICK, D.W., G. SANDRINI, and P. WILLIAMS. "Use of the Sustained Pain-Free Plus No Adverse Events Endpoint in Clinical Trials of Triptans in Acute Migraine." *CNS Drugs* 21, no. 1 (2007): 73–82.

DODICK, D.W., V.T. MARTIN, T. SMITH, and S. SILBERSTEIN. "Cardiovascular Tolerability and Safety of Triptans: A Review of Clinical Data." *Headache* 44, Supplement 1 (2004): S20–30.

EDMEADS, J. "Defining Response in Migraine: Which Endpoints Are Important?" *European Neurology* 53, Supplement 1 (2005): 22–28.

EVANS, R.W., S.J. TEPPER, R.E. SHAPIRO, C. SUN-EDELSTEIN, and G.E. TIETJEN. "The FDA Alert on Serotonin Syndrome with Use of Triptans Combined with Selective Serotonin Reuptake Inhibitors or Selective Serotonin-Norepinephrine Reuptake Inhibitors: American Headache Society Position Paper." *Headache* 50, no. 6 (2010): 1089–99.

FERRARI, M.D., P.J. GOADSBY, K.I. ROON, and R.B. LIPTON. "Triptans (serotonin, 5-HT1B/1D agonists) in Migraine: Detailed Results and Methods of a Meta-Analysis of 53 Trials." *Cephalalgia* 22, no. 8 (2002): 633–58.

FRANKLIN, G.M. "Opioids for Chronic Non-Cancer Pain: A Position Paper of the American Academy of Neurology." *Neurology* 83, no. 14 (2014): 1277–84.

GOADSBY, P.J., G. ZANCHIN et al. "Early vs. Non-Early Intervention in Acute Migraine — 'Act When Mild (AWM)'. A Double-Blind, Placebo-Controlled Trial of Almotriptan." *Cephalalgia*, 28, no. 4 (2008): 383–91.

KELMAN, L. "The Broad Treatment Expectations of Migraine Patients." *Journal of Headache Pain* 7, no. 6 (2006): 403–06.

KOTECHA, M.K., and B.D. SITES. "Pain Policy and Abuse of Prescription Opioids in the USA: A Cautionary Tale for Europe." *Anaesthesia* 68, no. 12 (2013): 1210–15.

LANTERI-MINET, M., H. ALLAIN, P.L. DRUAIS, G. MERIC, and S. TROY. "Evaluating Patient Satisfaction with Specific Migraine Therapy Based on Initial Treatment Expectations: The PAX Study." *Current Medical Research and Opinion* 26, no. 2 (2010): 465–72.

LODER, E., E. WEIZENBAUM, B. FRISHBERG, and S. SILBERSTEIN. "Choosing Wisely in Headache Medicine: The American Headache Society's List of Five Things Physicians and Patients Should Question." *Headache* 53, no. 10 (2013): 1651–59.

MESSALI, A.J., M. YANG et al. "Treatment Persistence and Switching in Triptan Users: A Systematic Literature Review." *Headache* 54, no. 7 (2014): 1120–30.

ORR, S.L., M. AUBE et al. "Canadian Headache Society Systematic Review and Recommendations on the Treatment of Migraine Pain in Emergency Settings." *Cephalalgia* 35, no. 3 (2014): 271–84

PRINGSHEIM, T., W. DAVENPORT et al. "Canadian Headache Society Guideline for Migraine Prophylaxis." *Canadian Journal of Neurological Sciences* 39, Supplement 2 (2012): S1–59.

PRYSE-PHILLIPS, W., M. AUBE et al. "A Clinical Study of Migraine Evolution." *Headache* 46, no. 10 (2014): 1480–86.

REVICKI, D.A., M. KIMEL et al. "Validation of the Revised Patient Perception of Migraine Questionnaire: Measuring Satisfaction with Acute Migraine Treatment." *Headache* 46, no. 2 (2006): 240–52.

SAPER, J.R., S. SILBERSTEIN, D. DODICK, and A. RAPOPORT. "DHE in the Pharmacotherapy of Migraine: Potential for a Larger Role." Headache 46 Suppl 4 (2006): S212-20.

TFELT-HANSEN, P.C., and P.J. KOEHLER. "History of the Use of Ergotamine and Dihydroergotamine in Migraine from 1906 and Onward." *Cephalalgia* 28, no. 8 (2008): 877–86.

TFELT-HANSEN, P.C., T. PIHL, A. HOUGAARD, and D.D. MITSIKOSTAS. "Drugs Targeting 5-Hydroxytryptamine Receptors in Acute Treatments of Migraine Attacks. A Review of New Drugs and New Administration Forms of Established Drugs." *Expert Opinion on Investigational Drugs* 23, no. 3 (2014): 375–85.

VALADE, D. "Early Treatment of Acute Migraine: New Evidence of Benefits." *Cephalalgia* 29, Supplement 3 (2009): 15–21.

VIANA, M., A.A. GENAZZANI, G. TERRAZZINO, G. NAPPI, and P.J. GOADSBY. "Triptan Nonresponders: Do They Exist and Who Are They?" *Cephalalgia* 33, no. 11 (2013): 891–96.

WENZEL, R.G., S. TEPPER, W.E. KORAB, and F. FREITAG. "Serotonin Syndrome Risks When Combining SSRI/SNRI Drugs and Triptans: Is the FDA's Alert Warranted?" *Annals of Pharmacotherapy* 42, no. 11 (2008): 1692–96.

WELLS, R.E., S.Y. MARKOWITZ et al. "Identifying the Factors Underlying Discontinuation of Triptans." *Headache* 54, no. 2 (2014): 278–89.

Chapter 8

AURORA, S.K., P. WINNER et al. "Onabotulinumtoxin A for Treatment of Chronic Migraine: Pooled

Analyses of the 56-Week PREEMPT Clinical Program." *Headache* 51, no. 9 (2011): 1358–73.

BLUMENFELD, A., S.D. SILBERSTEIN et al. "Method of Injection of Onabotulinumtoxin A for Chronic Migraine: A Safe, Well-Tolerated, and Effective Treatment Paradigm Based on the PREEMPT Clinical Program." *Headache* 50, no. 9 (2010): 1406–18.

BOGDANOV, V.B., S. MULTON et al. "Migraine Preventive Drugs Differentially Affect Cortical Spreading Depression in Rat." *Neurobiology of Disease* 41, no. 2 (2011): 430–35.

DIB, M. "Optimizing Prophylactic Treatment of Migraine: Subtypes and Patient Matching." *Therapeutics and Clinical Risk Management*, no. 5 (2008): 1061–78.

DIENER, H.C. "Acupuncture Prophylaxis of Migraine No Better Than Sham Acupuncture for Decreasing Frequency of Headaches." *Evidence-Based Medicine* 18, no. 1 (2013): 33–34.

EVANS, R.W., and M. LINDE. "Expert Opinion: Adherence to Prophylactic Migraine Medication." *Headache* 49, no. 7 (2009): 1054–58.

GOADSBY, P.J., T. BARTSCH, and D.W. DODICK "Occipital Nerve Stimulation for Headache: Mechanisms and Efficacy." *Headache* 48, no. 2 (2008): 313–18.

LINDE, K., G. ALLAIS et al. "Acupuncture for Migraine Prophylaxis." *Cochrane Database of Systematic Reviews* (1) (2009): CD001218.

MARTELLETTI, P., R.H. JENSEN et al. "Neuromodulation of Chronic Headaches: Position Statement from the European Headache Federation." *Journal of Headache Pain* 14 (2013): 86.

PICKETT, H., and J.C. BLACKWELL. "FPIN's Clinical Inquiries. Acupuncture for Migraine Headaches." *American Famimly Physician* 81, no.8 (2010): 1036–37.

PRINGSHEIM, T., W.J. DAVENPORT, and W.J. BECKER. "Prophylaxis of Migraine Headache." CMAJ 182, no. 7 (2010): E269–276.

SUN-EDELSTEIN, C., and A. MAUSKOP. "Foods and Supplements in the Management of Migraine Headaches." *Clinical Journal of Pain* 25, no. 5 (2009): 446–52.

YANG, C.P., M. H. CHANG et al. "Acupuncture Versus Topiramate in Chronic Migraine Prophylaxis: A Randomized Clinical Trial." *Cephalalgia* 31, no. 15 (2011): 1510–21.

RESOURCES

Migraine Québec: www.migrainequebec.com

Migraine Canada: www.migrainecanada.com

Dr. Elizabeth Leroux's royalties for books sold in French in Canada are donated to the Fonds pour la Migraine at the Fondation du CHUM.

IMAGE CREDITS

Also in the Your Health Series

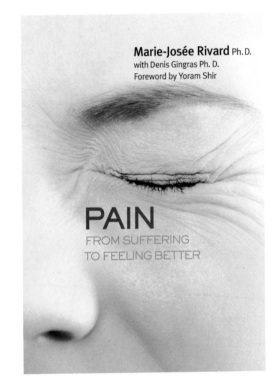

PAIN
From Suffering to Feeling Better
Marie-Josée Rivard, Ph.D.

Pain strikes all of us, but it becomes a recurring or constant condition for one in five people. For millions, young and old, it is a difficult, day-to-day reality, and many sufferers have been left feeling more frustrated and helpless than ever, despite medical advances.

Pain is a guide to understanding and treating all kinds of pain, and helping sufferers maintain hope for a normal life. In accessible chapters, this book explains how pain occurs at a fundamental level, both psychologically and physically, and what makes ordinary pain debilitating.

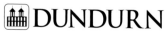